MW00571777

HOW AM I GONNA FIND A MAN IF I'M DEAD?

FANNY GAYNES

Morgin Press, Inc.
Wayne, PA
1994

MORGIN PRESS INC.
303 W. Lancaster Ave. #283
Wayne, PA 19087 U.S.A.

Gaynes, Fanny 1946-1993
How Am I Gonna Find A Man If I'm Dead? / Fanny Gaynes
p. cm.
ISBN 0-9630976-4-4

Library of Congress Cataloguing-in-Publishing Data
CIP 93-080044

MORGIN PRESS books are available at special discounts for bulk purchases, for sales promotions, premiums, fund-raising, or educational use. For details contact:
Special Sales Director
Morgin Press Inc.
303 W. Lancaster Ave. #283
Wayne PA.19087 U.S.A.

Cover Design: Izhar Zik & Barbara Solot. Graphics V, Philadelphia
Cover photograph: Robin Chin
Book Design and Layout: Julia Aureden
Editing: Mary Lowe Kennedy / Caslon, Inc.
Proofreader: Jennifer Baldino
Printed and Bound by: Maple-Vail Press Co.

First Edition
10 9 8 7 6 5 4 3 2

For my friends who know me,
and for Grace and Nicole so they will.

This is a true story. The places in this book are real, and the people are real, too – but some of them are in disguise. When you're dealing with cancer, opening up other kinds of wounds just doesn't seem necessary.

The treatment plans I describe are real as well. But there are a couple of important points to make about them.

First, I am *in no way* recommending any particular kind of therapy for a person with cancer. (After all, as you'll see, none of the ones I've tried has been a magic wand for me.) What I *do* recommend is that you ask a lot of questions, do a lot of reading and find out what your options are.

Second, the information I give about these programs is what I understood to be true *when I went into them.* Research continues, more results come in, and expert opinions change. Again, do that research.

And never lose hope.

F.G.

HOW AM I GONNA FIND A MAN IF I'M DEAD?

FANNY GAYNES

TABLE OF CONTENTS

INTRODUCTION

At forty-two, my Great-Great-Aunt Fay was told she had only six months to live. In keeping with an ancient Jewish tradition of changing your name in order to fool the Angel of Death, Great-Great-Aunt Fay became Chaya Bella. Aunt Chaya Bella, today, plays poker and waits for Willard Scott to wish her a happy 101st.

At forty-two, when I learned that breast cancer, diagnosed seven years earlier, had found its way to my lungs, I immediately vowed to change my name too. I even planned to clear out of L.A., with no forwarding address, to keep that Angel on her toes. But just in case these didn't do the trick, I would also endure the most aggressive treatment I could find at the time – an experimental bone-marrow transplant – which would literally take me to death's door in a last-ditch effort to save my life.

With transplants for breast cancer still so new, investigating my options was grueling, obsessive, relentless, lonely. Sifting through the rat's nest of conflicting views, small numbers, huge risks, and available programs – making an informed decision about something for which there is little information – was the most painful and exhilarating experience of my life. I was dying, yet, at the same time, I was an astronaut preparing to go to the moon.

Mine is the story I would like to have read when I was embarking on all of this: A model for leaving no stone unturned – in English rather than Medicalese. A tribute to friendship, family, support, great doctors, and the urgency of humor. A companion who's been there whom you don't have to talk to – and who, more importantly, doesn't talk back.

And mine is a story much less about dying than it is about coming alive. A true awakening: emotionally, spiritually, physically, sexually, with love and miracles, "accidents" and dreams – all the weird stuff that, until I'd been through it, I'd always referred to as "Hoogie Moogie."

It's a wonderful story. I know: I was there. It's for everyone – and especially for anyone in a medical crisis or who knows someone who is. For the thousands of women diagnosed with breast cancer every year, and all the rest who live in fear, knowing their chances of getting it sooner or later are better than one in nine. For the far too many women who've shocked me by telling me, too late, that their doctors never told them of their experimental options. You don't have to take the options – but you have a right to know you can.

My friends Steffie and Jimmy have a teenage daughter, Kate, who was diagnosed six years ago with an inoperable brain tumor and given six months to live. After scouring the world for the best medical treatment, they eventually settled on radiation. The day before Kate was to begin the treatment, a friend of Steffie's phoned to say she'd seen mention in a magazine of a doctor in another state doing experimental laser surgery for brain tumors. Steffie called his clinic and learned that Kate was eligible – so long as she had had *no* prior radiation treatment to the area of the tumor. The next day, instead of going for radiation, Kate went straight to the clinic. Six years later, she's tumor-free and kicking.

Now, this was a treatment that surely wouldn't work for everyone – or maybe even for very many – but it worked for *her*. And it's horrible to think about what might have happened had Kate received even one dose of radiation before learning about the laser program. One little radiation treatment – plus a program requirement that was very likely arbitrary, something the doctor had to adopt in order to get a grant – and the door could have slammed on a young girl's life.

If anything in my story helps one person the way Kate was helped by that woman's call, I'll know why it is – besides sunsets and shopping and sex – that I lived to tell it.

PART ONE

SOOTHING THE SAVAGE BREAST

I have this recurring dream. I'm flying in an airplane. The left wing falls off. The plane crashes. I survive the crash. But they lose my luggage.

One

❦

I wore a middy blouse, pigtails, and jeans to Dr. Weiner's. That way I couldn't possibly have a grown-up disease.

"I've a strangeness in my left breast," I said to the receptionist, having barged in without an appointment and unable, as yet, to use the word "lump."

"Don't tell me where, Jill," Weiner (Or Doctor, as he called himself, as in "Hi, Jill. This is Doctor.") said, as he felt.

"So how've you been, Doctor?"

"Enh-h-h-h," he whined.

"*That* bad?" I tried to keep the ball rolling.

"Enh-h-h-h. I'm surviving."

"D'ya find anything yet?" I asked, trying to sound casual.

"Nothing unusual. Maybe you better show me."

I showed him.

He said, "Uh-oh."

I almost threw up.

Then he suggested I see Dr. Klein, "the best breast specialist in the West."

On the way out, I thought about my checkup three months prior. Had the lump been there then? Had Doctor missed it? And if it wasn't there then, when did it come? What happens at that very exact moment when a lump becomes palpable? Is it like catching a cold – one minute you're fine, the next minute you're sneezing? Where was *I* and what was I doing in that instant when *mine* became palpable? Was I eating something? Maybe I was eating peas and one of the peas got stuck in my breast. Or walnuts. You always hear, "It was the size of a pea . . . the size of a walnut . . ." Shit, I'd had watermelon just last week.

Or maybe it happened during sex. Sex – that's it! And that's why Richard, my husband, found it instead of me. It had popped into palpability during a moment of passion. (Like a little erection. That'll teach *me*.) But how long had it been there? Had Richard actually felt it just as it decided to become a full-fledged lump? That would make it two weeks old. Or had he, too, missed it in earlier routine feel-ups? If so, are we talking weeks, months, years, all my life? And why am I sitting here trying to blame *them*? Where was I during all that time? Why the hell hadn't *I* found the lump?

Within fifteen minutes I was at Dr. Klein's.

"I've a strangeness in my left breast," I said to the receptionist, figuring the line had worked once. It worked again.

"Most of the women who come in here are sure they've got something wrong, but they don't. You're not one of them," Dr. Klein said.

I liked his style. He was seasoned and sweet and he knew how to laugh. At seventy-two, he looked fifty-five, but not in the L.A. face-lift way; he just seemed to have taken good care of himself.

And I liked his setup. Even though it was Beverly Hills, his office was modest and run by one woman, Flo, also in her seventies, with whom he'd obviously been working for years. At lunch, every day, they split "one water bagel and just a little cream cheese."

"I'm going to aspirate the lump," he went on, grabbing a needle the length of my leg. "If we get water, that means it's a cyst. And if it's a cyst, that means we're home free."

I prayed to the cyst gods and closed my eyes, amazed to discover the needle didn't hurt.

"Well," he said, a hundred years later, "just because we didn't get water doesn't necessarily mean we're in trouble. Eighty percent of these lumps are benign. But we'd better do a biopsy and find out for sure."

I took one of the deeper breaths of my thirty-five years and said, "O.K., then, let's get the show on the road."

"We can do it a week from next Thursday," he said.

"A week from next Thursday! That's almost two weeks!"

"I'm awfully sorry, but I'm booked straight through."

Having always had a problem with delayed gratification, I left and went directly to Baskin-Robbins.

Having always had a problem with delayed *reaction*, I burst into tears the moment I learned they were out of Jamoca Almond Fudge.

Barbara and I had been friends since age seven, when they moved her house from First Street to Sixth – a feat which never ceased to amaze me – and plopped it into the hole in the ground where I'd been playing for over a year. She and I used to play basketball every day at her house. And sleep over at each other's on alternate weekends. Once I even packed a typewriter case full of clothes and ran all seven houses away to hers, planning to live there forever. And now I remembered that somewhere in her twenties, Barbara had had a tumor removed that turned out to be benign. It was time to call Barbara and talk benign tumors.

It was so wonderful, hearing her voice. We talked for over an hour, about everything: Her marriage. My marriage. Therapy. Work. School. Fat. Biking. Running. Everything but benign tumors. I just couldn't get the "T" word out of my mouth.

After we said goodbye, I sat there clinging to the breezy calm covering the terror within. Having heard me hang up, my husband came into the room. "Listen," he said, "I'd appreciate it if you'd shorten those long-distance calls" – now, if he had just stopped there, but no – " 'cause otherwise I'll have to rip out the phone."

"Go ahead," I invited, more calmly than ever, partly because I didn't want to give him the satisfaction of seeing what his words did to me, and partly because I knew he was angry about something else. I MIGHT DIE. And then we'd really be talking long distance . . .

So he took out his anger, along with the phone and part of the wall, then left me in what remained of the room.

And I sat there. Just staring. Staring and rocking, trying like crazy to put terror on hold, not wanting to spend it unless it was called for, which surely it wouldn't be, since eighty percent of breast tumors are benign.

And I'd probably still be there, staring and rocking, if Richard hadn't come back to escalate things. I've blocked out the words, but we're talking pure rage. Knock-down, drag-out, primitive rage. Knocking down, dragging out every old issue in which we'd engaged. Sex – more specifically, the lack thereof; money – how do you define "work" that contributes to the "community"? And what about L.A., Jill? Couldn't you just *try* to like it?

The details are hazy. But the next thing I remember, Richard was saying those three little words he'd said so often:

"Get out, Jill!"

And I'd always figured that's what he meant (how was I to know he was begging *me* to beg to stay?). I'd also figured that's what I deserved – to be the one to "get out" if there were getting out to be done. After all, according to Mr. Perfecto, it was *I* who was the "depressed sack of shit" in this marriage. The Ice Maiden. Anger Woman. Selfish Bitch.

So, as always, I pulled out my little green suitcase and started to pack my T-shirts and books, thinking who'll get the stereo? Where will I go? I can't stay at Samantha's – she doesn't allow people to smoke in her house, maybe I should do a load of laundry first, shit, if this were Chicago, at least I'd have friends, or I'd live at the Y – did I say the Y? The *Y*! Oh my God, girl, get a grip.

And with that, I threw down my green bag and said those three little words that changed our lives:

"*You* pack, Fuckface!"

During the two weeks before the biopsy, there were several more fights. One was over a baked potato. Another was over an upside-down towel. But the best was one when I started to scream “Richard!” and instead out fell “Mother!” – which kept us from killing each other. We were laughing too hard.

Two

❦

Driving to the hospital, I thought back three months to my thirty-fifth birthday, when I'd broken my tooth on a piece of chicken. Boiled chicken. You know what that's like? That's like breaking your tooth on a piece of soup. I really felt awful about it. "I'm finished," I'd announced. "All washed up. Over the hill. Finito. Kaput." I could hardly imagine anything worse.

Now, heading for the biopsy, I wondered how many teeth I would trade . . .

Then I thought about the medicine Dr. Weiner had prescribed the year before, after some minor cervical surgery. Preventive medicine, "just so things stay good down there." Yellow, yucky, smelly goop, inserted three times a week for the rest of my life. For the rest of my life! I could hardly imagine anything worse.

Approaching the hospital, I wondered if I'd even need my next refill.

❧

If I'd known they were going to give me so many blood tests, I would've studied harder. And if I'd known Inspector Number Twelve was going to give me my mammogram, I would've run away.

"Right one first and don't scream when it's cold."

"Yes'm," I muttered sarcastically as she jammed my breast into a big steel vice and cranked a handle to tighten it up. "Oh my God!"

"Wouldn't hurt so much if you weren't so damn small."

When it was finally over, she did a Jekyll-and-Hyde. Sweet as anything, she patted me on the back and said, "Mammo looks good. Don't show nothing at all."

"Thanks," I said, almost skipping out of the room. "And I'm not all that small. In fact, I'm just right!"

Since the mammogram looked so good, I could now give the chest X-ray my undivided terror. Having smoked publicly since age fourteen, privately since twelve, I was always certain my number was up whenever there was occasion to X-ray my chest. That day I decided it was time to strike a bargain. If the X-ray didn't catch me, I'd quit; that was it.

The results of the chest X-ray wouldn't be in until the following day. That meant I had a busy night of smoking ahead. Not to mention eating and drinking (you have to stop at midnight before general anesthesia). Oh, yes, and someone came in to shave my breast. That was weird. And her name was Carey. So, of course, I took the opportunity to say, "I assume you're here to commit hairy, Carey!"

And she didn't laugh. Which made me feel lonely. So I stayed awake an extra hour . . . to have one last Mounds bar at 11:59.

❧

It was Richard who told me. I heard him, but not really.

Partly, I'm sure, because of the drugs, but mostly because, despite my terror, in my heart of hearts I never ever really believed it would be anything but benign.

I can't imagine what it would be like to have to tell someone you love they've got cancer. Or someone you don't love, for that matter. Malignant. *Malignant.* What a potent word. Thank God for the drugs. It took time to sink in. (I mean, I was so drugged, the bone scan that followed was fun.)

The next thing I knew, it was Friday morning. And there was Dr. Klein, sitting on my bed, his hands on my knees, which could only mean the tumor was still malignant. (Did I really believe it could change overnight? When I gave it some thought, the answer was yes.)

"First the good news," he said.

I lit up.

"The tests we did yesterday indicate the tumor is localized to the breast. That means we have a couple of choices." (Whatcha mean *we*? And whatcha mean *choices*? Don't you know you're dealing with a terminal ambivalent here?)

"We can perform a lumpectomy; that is, remove the tumor and surrounding tissue, which, in essence, the biopsy has already accomplished. And then you'd have radiation treatments for six weeks, and, at the end of those treatments, a radiation implant, which would stay in for about two days, kind of like a booster shot, just to make sure."

"Uh-huh," I said, shaking and hearing about every third word.

"Or we could perform a modified radical mastectomy, where we remove the breast and axillary lymph nodes, but not the pectoral muscles."

I was starting to get queasy, but I let him continue.

"If you decide to go for the mastectomy, we could do it this coming Monday. After that, I'm leaving town for three weeks, so we could do it when I come back."

He could see by my face that this was a lot to absorb.

"Look," he said, "you can take some time and think this thing out. But from the little I know about you, if you opt for the mastectomy, you're not going to want to wait three weeks. Why don't I schedule you for Monday? If you haven't reached a decision by then, or if you've decided to go the lumpectomy route, we'll cancel. How's that?"

"From the little you know of me, you know me well. Thanks," I said, as I gave him a hug.

"Meanwhile, I suggest you check out for the weekend and celebrate."

"Celebrate!?"

He turned purple. "I'm sorry. It's the Fourth of July."

The doctor left and I found myself drifting. To July 12, 1961. My fifteenth year. I remember what I was wearing (I always remember significant dates by how I covered my body): emerald-green rayonette clam diggers and matching emerald-green jacket that I had borrowed from Steffie Wolff, who'd borrowed-from-and-never-returned-them-to Lisa Rothberg, who'd worked-at-and-stolen-them-from Saks. All this to look casually perfect for Dale Lurie's Sweet Sixteen. And lucky thing, because Rolla Herman phoned the party to see if I wanted to be fixed up with Bruce Fine – that night, right after the party. This would be my first blind date. Of course I said yes; a vision in emerald, how could I miss?

I felt sorry for Bruce the minute I saw him. He was

gorgeous. With hair on his chest. I mean, he was a man. Nineteen; about to start his second year of college – what would he want with schleppy little me? And I'm talking MAN. I remember sitting across from him at the end of the evening and noticing, in the light of the heat lamp at Billy's Delicatessen, that he'd actually grown a beard during our date. I'd never seen anything like *this* before, not on anyone *I* hung around with. Again feeling total pity for this person, I thought, *I bet he can't wait to get me home.*

And I was right. He *couldn't* wait to get me home – so he could kiss me and ask me out for the next night. Well, that was it. I was totally in love.

We saw each other every minute for the rest of the summer, and on weekends once he went away to school. Besides being gorgeous, he was kind and gentle and sensitive and funny. And very bright. An absolutely perfect boyfriend for someone fifteen who didn't know what she was doing.

One day, near the end of that first summer, we were sitting in my family room, close together on my mother's stiff grey couch. The phone rang and Bruce picked it up. As he handed it to me, his forearm sort of brushed against my left breast. (I was wearing an emerald-green, round-collared, nubby blouse, a Dacron poly-filled lightly padded bra, and some of the ugliest plaid Bermuda shorts ever seen.) I took the phone and made the conversation as brief as possible. Then I excused myself, went to the bathroom, and cried.

You might think I was teary because I was moved by Bruce's touching my breast. But that had never happened before. And I know this is going to be a tough one to swallow, but I was upset because I felt I'd been used. *Upset?*

I was devastated. Maybe, just maybe, he had brushed me by accident. But, somehow, it seemed he had done it on purpose – copped a feel without my knowing. And I hated feeling the fool. I can't believe that's how I was feeling –but that's *how* I was feeling. And *that*, as far as I was concerned, was my introduction to petting above the waist.

I eventually stopped crying and came back to the couch. We never discussed it. (Discussed *what*? In looking back, it's possible he didn't even know he'd done it. God, how could anything so simple have caused so much pain?)

Later that summer, we got around to the real thing – at least when it came to petting above the waist. And below for that matter. My memories are delicious: very tender, very sweet, and incredibly exciting. All the wonderful stuff you do when you're into doing "everything but." Imagine this foreplay in grown-up life lasting many years.

And now, twenty years later, as I lay in my hospital bed wondering whether to sacrifice my left breast, I remembered the time in early September of '61 when Bruce was leaving to go back to school. I was shaking all over, I was so upset at saying goodbye. We'd been hugging and kissing and snuggling and Bruce had been saying goodbye to my parts. He kissed my fingers and said goodbye. Then my nose and my eyes and my lips and my ears. After my ears, he came to my breasts.

"So long, Righty," he said to the right one. "Lefty, I'm gonna miss you," he said to the other.

As I lay there thinking of this wonderful man with whom I'd first discovered the pleasures of my breasts, I felt that, if I decided to have a mastectomy, I wanted him to come say so long to Lefty.

Three

❦

My mother was sitting in her clenched position, her short-sleeved, shivering, freckled arms pretzeled across her breasts. My father was sitting next to her in his Daddy's-here-everything'll-be-fine attitude. And I was lying on my hospital bed wondering how I'd moved so quickly from "will I love" to "will I live."

My mastectomy was twenty-four hours away.

I caught a glimpse of my father trying to yawn, the way he did when he was having trouble taking a deep breath – which made him even more conscious of trying to catch his breath – which made him even shorter of breath. I held my own breath, waiting for him to breathe – which made me short of breath – which made me try to yawn. We caught each other at it and laughed, which got us breathing again. Relieved, my dad took a nap in the palm of his hand. And I studied the scar on his forehead.

The scar reminded me of a continuing story he used to

tell me when I was little – "The Case of the Bashed-In Head." I have no memory of the story itself, but I'll never forget the thrill of the time we spent together in the telling. It hardly mattered what he was saying, just that he was saying it to me alone. It was *our* story, *our* secret.

When I was in my early teens, he told me another secret: As long as he could remember, he'd had a fantasy of crashing through windows. There was no particular emotion attached; he simply wanted to smash through glass. In later years, when I'd be with my family and see something I wanted in the window of a store that was closed, I'd nudge my dad and quietly say, "Looks like a job for Glass Man."

In my early thirties, "The Case of the Bashed-In Head" came back to haunt me. It was two months after I'd gotten married and moved to L.A. My parents had come out from Detroit for their winter vacation. On their second day there, my father-in-law unexpectedly died and my mother and father, who barely knew their recently acquired family, were sucked right into the storm.

The evening after the funeral we were all at my sister-in-law's, alternately commiserating and eating. My parents were about to leave for Palm Springs, where they planned to resume their vacation. At the last minute my father realized he'd forgotten to take his blood-pressure pills. He walked through the living room to the backyard, where there was some bottled water on a picnic table, and took his pills. I don't know who closed the sliding door my father had opened to get to the backyard – maybe he did it himself – but seconds later, I heard a huge thud and looked up to see him crash back through it, shattering the glass.

My mother was in the bathroom. She heard the crash and, somehow, understood exactly what had happened. She ran out, took one look at my father, blood gushing from his head, and screamed, "I knew it, I knew it!" She turned around and went back into the bathroom. My brother-in-law and I took my father to the hospital, where – five agonizing hours later – his blood pressure finally lowered enough so he could be given 200 stitches. While we waited, the image of my father walking through glass became a permanent slide in the carousel of my mind. Over and over I would see the image, eyes closed, eyes open, waking, sleeping, it didn't matter. And each time I'd see it, I'd find myself thinking that he had written the final chapter of "The Case of the Bashed-In Head."

Now, as I lay in my hospital bed, I wondered: Was that really a self-fulfilling prophecy? And if it was, if my father could do *that* to himself, could *I* have possibly caused *this*?

No! I'd always figured I'd be hit by a truck – the day after I'd found "true happiness," of course – *that's* how I'd go. On the other hand, I'd certainly had thoughts about "getting" cancer, but was *I* any more cancer-phobic than average? Surely not – especially if you took as a clue my cursory, once-every-few-months, standing-in-the-shower breast self-exams. Besides, if thinking about cancer *causes* cancer, then why doesn't everyone have it? Phew. Relieved to have figured *that* one out, I lay back and closed my eyes to nap.

But it didn't work. I could shut my eyes, but not my mind. All of my logic drained from me as I carried myself further inside to the answer I never really wanted to know. My deep-down truth, when I really got to it, was – without a doubt – I blamed myself. In my very rational grown-up brain, I knew I couldn't have made this happen. But deep, deep down in that primitive place where I always remain a child – I believed that when something bad happened, it was *always* my fault.

It was my fault my father walked through that door. *My* fault. If only I hadn't married Richard. If only I hadn't moved to L.A. If only I hadn't suggested they come . . . The day after the accident, I told Richard I wanted us to move back to Detroit and live with my parents so I could monitor my father for the rest of his life.

As I watched him napping away in the palm of his hand, I suddenly realized that until that moment, I'd never even remotely considered the thought that *he* could outlive *me*. In the strangest mixture of grief and relief, I comforted myself with the possibility of never having to deal with my father's death.

As I watched my dad with his head in his hand, I also flashed on something else – me, at age five, waking to find his very same hand, cold and trembling, on my little forehead.

"It worked. It worked," he muttered.

"What worked, Daddy?"

"Nothing, sweetheart." By now he was beaming. "Just get some rest."

Later, I heard him confess to my grandma, "I swore off chocolate so the fever would break."

No wonder my father was napping away. Napping away his pain. I ached for him as I finally realized that deep, deep down in that primitive place where *he* always remained a child, my man/child/daddy was just like me – he "knew" my cancer was all his fault.

As if he'd overheard my thoughts, my father snapped awake, lit a cigarette and offered me one. I lit it with my butane lighter that bore the message "Go with the flow." As

I inhaled, it came to me – the other side of believing it's all your fault is believing you can fix it. But where to start? Remembering the promise I'd made to myself a few days before when they'd X-rayed my chest, I announced to my dad, "That does it. I'm quitting."

"Your job?"

"No, smoking," I said, inhaling more deeply, more passionately than ever. "At midnight."

Melodramatically, my dad blew a smoke ring. And then another, right through the first. He watched them disappear as he said, "O.K., then me too. We'll have a pact."

"A pact," I gulped, knowing we'd just irrevocably quit – feeling in that totally irrational, unspeakable way, we each had the power to keep the other alive.

❧

Waiting. Wondering. And watching myself, watching my parents watching me, watching them waiting, and wondering. The longest day.

Like the day I waited for Danny Stone to return from school after three months away. A slow-motion day . . . long walks, long lunch, a long nap . . . and just plain longing. I even took the longest bath, shaving each leg one hair at a time, trying to remember where his body would meet mine when we'd wrap ourselves around each other and surrender to the heat of our nineteen-year-old flesh – through all of our clothes.

I was still in the bath when the doorbell rang. Danny was early. I couldn't believe it. There was his voice, right here in my house, and here was my body, right there in the tub. Forever had come and I wasn't ready. Quickly, I pushed myself up out of the water – and was smitten by a pain so sharp I slid right back down.

I felt as if I'd been shot in the heart. The tiniest breath felt like the stab of a knife. If I breathed any deeper I knew I would die. I couldn't scream for help; it took too much breath. So I sat there trying to breathe over the knife with the shortest bare minimum breaths I could find. But the pain began to spread to my arms. Oh, my God – a heart attack.

The door was locked. I still couldn't scream. By the time my mother got through charming Danny and began to wonder about me, I would just be tragic history. There was nothing I could do, so I surrendered to a God I wasn't even certain I believed in yet, while sweat coated any parts of my body that had started to dry. I tried to listen for the last words I would ever hear from Danny – something about " . . . no, thanks, milk'll be fine" – and I thought about how unfair things were. Here I was, nineteen and dying, dying in the tub. Danny would finally see me nude. But I would never see him. Ever.

That was the thought that got me crying. Which made me realize I was breathing more deeply. Which made me realize the knife was gone. Which made me realize I'd probably just had my first full-fledged anxiety attack.

Phew. Not a heart attack after all. Just an attack of the heart.

❧

Still waiting and wondering, I looked at my parents. They were still watching. I looked at my watch. Three minutes had whizzed on by. How many more "longest days" would I have to remember to get through *this* longest day? How many more sets of "three minutes" until midnight? Midnight, when they'd give me a pill and I'd go to sleep, till they woke me up to put me to sleep . . .

Still ticking. 5:55. Enter Esther. Tall – thin – dark – beautiful. Carefully dressed for aerobics, though her blazing red nails suggested it was just a disguise. Wardrobe and makeup had done their job. Esther was a cancer survivor, mid-thirties. A walking, talking, jumping-jacking, living, breathing health-o-gram.

"You've gotta be Esther," I screamed, just knowing this was the person who matched the voice that had given me so much comfort on the phone. "Mom, Dad – wake up, Dad – meet Esther!"

My doctor had given me Esther's number and we had met over the phone. She was clever, sweet, funny and cheery, but she had enough of an edge not to come off like a perky little Barbie doll. Uplifting and believable . . . a nice combination. And now she'd come to meet me in person in order to wish me luck on my surgery and show me her reconstructed breast.

My dad said hello and went back to sleep.

Esther didn't waste any time. As my father slept, she lifted her sweatshirt, proudly displaying her breasts for my mother and me to examine. I'd expected the reconstructed one to look more like the real one. It was rounder, but it still looked pretty good. My mother started shooting questions at Esther. How long did she wait after the mastectomy? Who was her doctor? Any complications? Any regrets? I closed my eyes and let Esther take over, allowing my thoughts to drown out their talk.

With her arrival, I found I needed to go over my decision – again. Again and again. I had made it so fast, in two-and-a-half days, I had to keep checking to make sure it still fit.

I had taken my first impulse – "Get it out of here, take

my breast, take as much as you have to, take more" – and filtered its visceral and emotional content through journals, texts, doctors, hotlines, friends, family and, ultimately, me. I had found out as much as I could about my family history, my particular type of tumor and my statistical chances for survival, based on the most current studies. There were studies of people with my size and type of tumor that indicated no significant difference in survival rates between those who'd had mastectomies with no further treatment and those who'd had lumpectomies with follow-up radiation. In 1981, however, those studies were only five years old, while the studies involving just mastectomies, with and without adjuvant chemotherapy, were already ten years old. Where were the lumpectomy people going to be in another five or ten years? Where was *I* going to be if I were one of them? I asked myself how I would feel if I were around for headlines that said "Mastectomy Not Necessary, No Matter Who, Where, Why, What Size or Type of Tumor."

I decided if I were alive to read a headline like that, I'd be more than thrilled for us all. I had to base my choice on the moment in medical history when all of this was happening. Happening to me – ME. I had to give myself the best possible shot.

I had been put to the test. And I passed.

I didn't want to die.

For a moment, I wondered about people who were more concerned with the loss of their breasts than the loss of their lives. I couldn't imagine feeling that way. Then I realized that this was a new me, quite different from the me I was used to. The old me was Little Ms. Immediate Gratification. The veritable Queen of Repression. Why was I suddenly willing and able to go straight to the real problem, straight to the cancer, straight to the forest, right through the trees?

My thoughts seemed too logical, too rational, too sound, and therefore, I figured, since I'd never in my life been logical, rational or close to sound, I was probably going insane. Or maybe I was just faking "normal," so that God – if there *was* one – would stop punishing me. Like the time I fake-ate lima beans, chewing, then spitting them into my napkin and stuffing them in pockets, so my mother would give me dessert.

Dessert, please. Mother? God? Waiter? Oh-h, waiter-r-r? Birthday cake, please. When I'm seventy-five.

I opened my eyes to ask my mother if she ever knew about those beans, but she was still firing away at Esther – "Did it hurt? Is it tender? Do you have any feeling?" She was still focusing on the loss of my breast.

Oh my God. My breast. Tomorrow, it would be gone. Forever. Esther was there to show us I could "buy" a new one. But that's not the same – that's not ME. The part of me they call my breast would never be there again, ever. My logical, rational thoughts were disappearing and being replaced by an overwhelming wave of nausea. I couldn't breathe. The room was spinning. *Breathe, Jill. Just breathe.* It's O.K.. Just breathe. No. If I breathe, I'll feel. If I feel, I'll cry. If I cry, I'll . . . Stop protecting THEM already. Start protecting YOU. Get it out. Breathe it out. Shout it out. Scream it out. Do something, Mother. Help me, Mother. Don't just sit there frozen in fear – read my mind, just this once. Please. Help me. I'm your daughter. I'm your baby. I need you. Now. Please. Now. Say something, now. Anything, now. Say, "Breathe, Baby, breathe." Say, "It's O.K." Say,

"Mommy's here." Tell me you love me. Tell me the doctor's not going to hurt me. Oh, God, Mother, don't make me mother *myself*. Not *now*. Not today. Not today. It's so clear, in this moment, as I watch you with Esther, chatting away – as I watch me with *me*, struggling to find the game in my mind that'll take me away, a joke, a rhyme, some comic relief, anything, please – *my God* – we are the same. After all, in the end, is there any real difference between clenching and cartwheels?

I slid off the bed and into the bathroom. I sat for a while, legs crossed, head down, on the floor, with the door slightly cracked so I could see *them*, but they couldn't see *me*. Esther and my mother were discussing reconstructed nipples. Almost against my will, I listened.

" . . . they grafted some skin from my upper thigh," Esther was explaining, "although they can also use some dark skin from the labia. They used to save the old nipple and graft it onto the reconstructed breast, but they found out it's risky because sometimes there are hidden cancer cells in the ducts of the old nipple."

Someone above, in charge of the strings that controlled my mother's marionette face, was pulling them now, more tightly than ever. So tightly they finally snapped. So tightly that finally her face fell and her voice cracked as she whispered to Esther, "I wish I could give her mine."

When the surgery finally came, I missed it – pretty much, anyway – thanks to drugs. But I did succeed in making myself a minor legend in the operating room.

Just before we got started, for some reason one of the

nurses asked if I were Russian. I am, by descent, but . . .

"No," I told her. "I'm not in any hurry. Just tell the doctor to take his time and do it right."

They still tell the story.

❧

The first few days after the surgery were a blur of visitors, phone calls, flowers, love, and those three little words I said to the doctor when he came every day to check my incision – "I can't look."

"You'll look when you're ready," he always assured me.

Ready for what? *Look* for what? How can you look for something that's not there? Where was my breast now, anyway? Was it stored in the hospital with all the other breasts? In the breast nursery perhaps? Could I visit it? Instead of babies in a nursery sucking bottles, I pictured breasts in a nursery screaming, "This sucks!"

When I finally looked, about four days in, I heard myself squeaking at the top of my throat, "Nice job, Doctor, really, nice job." (So typical of me, at a moment like this, when the nausea was boxing its way through my pipes, to reassure the doctor.)

A few days later, when Dr. Klein told me I was healing nicely and ready to go home, I was so excited I hopped out of bed and started to pack all the presents my friends had brought me, including a beautiful white toy horse I'd been wanting to ride off into the night. As I combed his mane with my non-packing hand, Dr. Klein's eyelids lowered. So did his voice. "The path report from the lymph node dissection came in a while ago."

I tucked my head into the horse's neck and waited for the ax to fall.

"Of the thirty lymph nodes they removed, five showed

evidence of cancer."

"What does that mean?" I asked, yanking on the horse's reins.

"Even though there's no technological evidence of spread outside the breast, when there's axillary lymph node involvement we treat as if there's the possibility of microscopic spread."

"And what does *that* mean?" My voice cracked.

"A year of chemotherapy."

My grip on the reins tightened until my fingernails cut the palm of my hand.

"Giddy up, Horsey."

Four

❦

Bandaged like a mummy from my waist to my neck, I checked out of the hospital with Mindy, my younger sister by eleven-and-a-half years. Anticipating a civilian-clothing fashion problem, Mindy surprised me with a wonderful gift – a really neat blouse with a high-collar neck that not only covered the entire bandage, but also hid my missing breast (no easy feat, hiding something that's not there).

Thanks to Mindy, I left the hospital feeling beautiful and very much alive. So alive I let no one forget it, insisting on celebrating – frantically, for hours. First, some shopping . . . at a lingerie store (was I in denial or merely insane?). Next, out to lunch and a matinee of the play *I'm Getting My Act Together and Taking It on the Road*. After that, dinner at my favorite seafood restaurant, right on the ocean. And finally, believe it or not, drinks and dancing at a country-western bar. Richard watched.

When we finally got home, I went straight to my answering machine to see if someone had left me a message that could possibly change my life. Like "Hi, Jill, Dr. Klein here. Just kidding about your nodes."

There were two messages: one from my psychotherapist's secretary, the other a response to an ad I'd been running to do freelance advertising copy. What timing, I thought. Work would help get my mind off things.

What timing was right. When I returned the work call, first thing in the morning, I learned it was Frederick's of Hollywood looking for a writer to promote their black lace, red-trimmed super-stuffer bra. I burst into tears and returned the call to my therapist's office, praying she'd be able to see me right away. This, however, was out of the question. The secretary had called to tell me that, while I was in the hospital, "you see, there was this accident."

My therapist was dead.

Despite these blows, coming to terms with my reshaped self was easier than I might have expected. One thing that helped, paradoxically, was my innate low level of confidence; I'd never expected anybody to love me for my looks anyway, and subtracting a breast didn't make things any worse.

Another thing that helped — a lot, it must be said — was Richard, my husband. Far from resenting my loss of a breast, he made it plain that he still found me quite attractive, even going so far as to insist on taking pictures of me topless.

And a third source of strength came from deep inside me. It turned out that, in matters of appearance versus health, I had a strong sense of priorities. These led me to decide against a breast implant for two big reasons: First, I felt strongly against doing anything *non-essential* to my body. And second, I had no sense of being "incomplete" without a breast – quite the contrary, I didn't want to feel even partly artificial in confronting the world. My attitude, I found, was: "*This* is me *now*."

So certain was I that when Dr. Klein advised me, during post-surgery checkups, about what kind of prosthesis I could get and where – just the simple on-with-the-bra type – my response was: "Thanks, but I doubt that I'll rush into anything." And that led to yet more self-discovery, because when he finally took the stitches out, I found myself heading right out to the Nearly Me store to buy one. Oh, well.

❧

Shopping for an oncologist to oversee my chemotherapy was harder than shopping for a used car. The first one I found had this to say when I mentioned a cancer article in *The New England Journal of Medicine:* "My advice to you – don't read." The second doctor at least asked the right questions; trouble was, he asked the wrong party – "So when did we discover the lump, Richard?" And when a third doctor whisked me through his overly decorated Beverly Hills office past "those wonderful nurses who draw the fastest blood in the West . . . and you'll wait hours for test results in a clinic setting, whereas we're committed to turning your blood over in five minutes or less," I waited for him to add: "Sign up now and get a free bamboo steamer."

Thank God I had the presence of mind to keep looking. I knew there had to be something more. And I found it, at UCLA, when a tall, dark doctor with soothing blue eyes walked into the examining room and immediately rearranged the seating so he would be interviewing *me*, not Richard. When this same gentle man, named Charles Mann, asked me all the right questions – questions that went to the core of my being, like "What's your reason for living?" – my heart began to pound. When he spoke to me in English instead of Medicalese, when he examined me with human hands, when he asked Richard to leave and looked me straight in the eyes and said, "Now, is there anything you'd like to tell me that you couldn't say in front of your husband?" – I knew I was home.

❧

With the job of finding a doctor completed, I could now devote full energy to my terror of chemotherapy, which would start in another week. Would there be a taste? Would there be a smell? Would I feel the toxins coursing through my veins? Would I puke my guts out? Barf my hair off? Lose eighty pounds? Be exhausted? Be depressed? Or would I be Ali McGraw in *Love Story*, brave and jokeful till the end? (THE END? *What* end?)

One afternoon, in a rare moment when I *wasn't* obsessing on the mysteries of chemotherapy, when for the first time since diagnosis I was actually relaxing, swinging in my hammock, reading a book, loving the garden, grateful for life on a gorgeous summer day – the phone rang.

I flew into the house and picked it up. Big mistake.

"Hi, Jill. My name's Phyllis Wunderkind. I'm a cousin of your mother-in-law and I hear we're members of the same sorority."

Puh-leeze, I thought, and responded: "Yeah, Theta Beta Titless."

Ignoring my sarcasm, she barreled ahead, bombarding me with the grim, gross story of her own mastectomy and chemotherapy. To put it mildly, things hadn't gone well. "The doctors warned me of all the side effects. I've had them *all.* And ones they never even dreamed of. They said I'd lose my hair, blah blah blah, but they never told me yada yada . . ."

There was no dialogue. Only monologue – nonstop and ad nauseam. Unable to get in even one word to stop her, I listened helplessly to the endless bad news and found myself growing dizzy and nauseous.

After forty-five minutes, this lunatic finally stopped talking about herself and directed a question to me. "How tall are you?" she asked. "You know they determine your dosage by size."

"Five-feet-four," I responded, then politely, and only God knows why, asked *her*, "And how tall are *you*?"

"Well . . ." She hesitated. "I used to be five-three, but now I'm five-one."

Oh no! I thought. Not *that* too!

❧

Thanks to Phyllis Wunderkind, my final days before chemotherapy were nothing short of excruciating. To my own obsessive fantasies were added visions of each and every one of her horrific side effects, now familiar to me in lurid detail. Knowing she was neurotic, I prayed that she had somehow made those stories up. But maybe the *chemo* had made her crazy; maybe I, too, would soon sport a demented mind.

Oh, how I wanted her stricken from my record, her memories erased forever from my mind. But I wasn't in the mood for a frontal lobotomy, so I looked in the yellow pages for the next best thing.

Duane Harvey, hypnotherapist, was a teeny bit on the

hokey side, but I was willing to do the Hokey Pokey. Anything to get back to square one before beginning chemo. Duane wore a lot of polyester. I could've counted backward from one hundred to zero much more easily if only he'd worn cotton.

I also found a new psychotherapist, Penelope. She wore cotton. And probably saved my life.

After a marathon week of hypnotherapy and psychotherapy, I went off to chemotherapy shaking like a kitten about to be spayed. Upon my doctor's advice, I smoked marijuana to help prevent nausea. Upon my hypnotherapist's advice, I pictured a chalkboard on which I wrote "nausea," then pictured an eraser wiping it away. Upon my psychotherapist's advice, I visualized warm, healing ocean water entering my veins through the needle with which I received my first drugs.

And upon my husband's advice, I aimed for the big bucket he held for me a few hours later – and puked my guts out.

Time, over the next year, was a blur of therapies – chemo, psycho, and polyester-hypno. In the chemotherapy I gained twenty pounds. In the psychotherapy I tried to learn why. In the hypnotherapy I tried to control it. And in my spare time I gained another twenty-five, finally deciding that only dying people don't gain weight.

I also decided to change my life, with a view to minimizing the demands I made on myself so I would have more energy for the physical battle. Also, as we say, I wanted to learn to smell the roses.

I needed to make these changes, however, in a style that was familiar. So, frenetically, I set out to become unfrenetic. Compulsively, I attempted to "decompulse." And obsessively, I labored at unobsessing. What a joke.

My first freelance advertising assignment offered a test for the new me: five radio spots for a jewelry store with diamond mines in South America, offices in Sri Lanka and diamond-cutting facilities in Israel. I thought to myself, this place is really classy; I'd better not do my usual funny stuff (for which I'd acquired a handsome reputation). Something *pretty* seemed more in order here. Besides, being funny is hard work and, since I'd always tended to overachieve, here was my chance to be an underachiever.

To prepare for the underachievement, I combed the city for days on end, collecting books on the history and folklore of gems. I read and read till my eyes were Slinkys, well into the night, spending more time trying to be serious or just "cute" than I'd ever spent trying to be funny.

One day, when I'd fallen asleep over the history and lore of the Hapsburg Tiara, I had the most ridiculous dream — the Brady Bunch was performing in concert. What were they singing? "I've Got to Be Me."

I awakened laughing and said to myself, "It's O.K. to be funny. That's *you.* Just don't work so hard at it." Then I threw down the books, grabbed a bucket of popcorn, flew to the typewriter and surprised myself with five of the easiest, breeziest, and funniest spots I'd ever written. Ah-ha, so the lesson: Be yourself.

Now all I had to do was stay alive to find out who that was.

My skin was yellow. My tastebuds were metal. I'd gained thirty percent of my original weight and lost fifty percent of my original hair (which I tried to replace at Ziggy's, the famous Hollywood wigmaker, where I was squeezed in for a fitting between Cheech and Chong – Cheech, Jill, Chong – which makes a better story than the wig I never wore).

Despite all this, I felt lighter than ever as I hopped out of bed – after two groggy days – from my final course of chemo. I followed the smell of fresh cappuccino into the kitchen, where Richard was sitting next to my cup, with a rose and a letter, one in each hand. I hugged him, smelled the rose and ripped right into the letter.

Oh, my God . . . it was notification that I'd won first place for "humorous radio" in one of the world's most prestigious competitions, the International Broadcasting Awards. *First place* for one of the spots that had been an experiment in underachieving and, ultimately, a lesson in being myself. What a wonderful end-of-chemo message: Be yourself. And win.

"C'mon," Richard said. "We're meeting Murray at Zucky's Delicatessen. He wants to celebrate your award." A cross between Alan Alda, Woody Allen, Mickey Mouse and a fox, Murray had been my friend since we worked together in a Chicago ad agency. He's brilliant, but so slow and preoccupied you could die. And with a dark sense of humor that had already helped lift me through this ghastly time as chemotherapy ate at my body and a bad marriage ate at my soul.

Now, there we were at Zucky's Deli, allegedly celebrating my radio award when, in the middle of my bagel, a man with a bugle approached the table and said, "Are you Jill?" Then he played a fanfare and shouted, for all the diners to hear:

"Ladies and gentlemen, we are not here to celebrate Jill's birthday. We are not here to celebrate her anniversary. No, ladies and gentlemen, we're here today" – more fanfare while I waited to be embarrassed about my award – "to celebrate the end of Jill's cheeeeee-m-oh-h-h-ther-r-r-r-apy . . ."

An unbearable song followed – with lyrics by Murray – while a mortified restaurant looked my way as I slid under the table, losing my bagel to prolonged laughter and my first hot flash – the *one* side effect from chemotherapy Phyllis Wunderkind failed to mention.

Five

❦

My re-entry into the real world was smooth and rocky, concomitantly. Like life. Smooth was the job I created for myself as an eight-month-a-year copywriter at a major agency, with full staff benefits including vacation, which, with holidays and all, whittled it down to seven months. Rocky was my marriage, which ultimately exploded at a joint therapy session when Richard admitted he'd rather I leave him than die on him – so I did. And proceeded to lose 240 pounds (40 of them mine).

Moving out of our home in Santa Monica to an apartment closer to downtown L.A., I made new friends and started living a less stressed, more honest, actually enjoyable life. In my time off, I'd hang out in L.A., or rent a place to write or just play in the mountains, at the ocean, even in Europe. And I hooked up with some composers. Started doing lyrics. Actually sold some songs.

My first lover, after the marriage ended, was a man

from San Diego who'd lost a leg to cancer. Our mutual asymmetry created a balance the likes of which I'd never known. Right from the start, without saying a word, we both understood, making passionate love to the parts of each other that were no longer there. My mastectomy, which is actually quite sweet (a very faint scar in the shape of a smile), had always hurt to the slightest touch. Now, as my lover so knowingly touched it, not only was there no pain, but I actually felt more sexual sensation – more excitement – than ever before. In fact, it was as if my breast were still there, but more sensitive than ever.

My first new girlfriend, post-marriage, shared with me a different kind of understanding. We met in a client session when I was just back from a trip to Europe, jet-lagged and certainly not up for the gig. The client, who was frighteningly serious about the product – an insipid doll named Rainbow Brite – was staring at me with empty eyes as I presented the commercial we were trying to sell, featuring an incredibly syrupy song written by me. As I heard it dripping out of my mouth, I became so embarrassed at being responsible for such drivel, and so uncomfortable with the silence of my client, that I moved into falsetto, raised my arms and beckoned the room, in lounge-lizard style: "*Eh-h-h*-vry-body!" Harriet was the only one who got the joke, her laughter falling on dead faces. On the way out of the meeting she pulled me aside and said, "Drink?" To which I responded, "Right away."

A half hour into our margaritas, Harriet and I knew more about each other than we did about ourselves – although I hadn't yet mentioned my cancer. As I was taking her through my pictures from Europe, we came across one of me on a nude beach. I grabbed it away quickly, announcing, "I'm not sure I'm ready for you to see *that.*" Harriet looked so puzzled that I reconsidered and said, "O.K., but I need to edit it just a little." Then I covered my thighs in the picture, and let her see the rest of it.

Harriet looked and looked, and finally said, sadly: "Oh, you've had a mastectomy." Which caught me completely off guard, since the last thing I'd been thinking about was hiding my not-there-anyway breast. No, I was truly hiding my too-much-there thighs. When I realized how ridiculous I was being from the waist down, yet how natural I was being from the waist up, I burst into laughter. Then I burst into tears.

We talked all about it. Inside and out. Four margaritas later, I blurted, "Are you sure you want to be friends with someone who has cancer?" She looked at me like I was crazy.

The next night, when we were watching a movie and I got a headache and was certain my cancer had metastasized to my brain, I think Harriet began to understand.

PART TWO

OUT OF THE TUNNEL INTO THE NIGHT

Six

❦

Seven-and-a-half years since my diagnosis. January 5, 1989. A darkened studio in Hollywood, California. Dr. Barbie (the doll) struts across the screen, demo-ing her stethoscope to the children of America, music blaring, voices singing her theme song – "We Girls Can Do Anything." I contain my disdain for that little plastic bitch – I mean that sweet little blonde role model who pays my bills. We're almost done. Maybe ten more minutes; then the commercial will be mixed and ready to ship, and I'll be out of there for four whole months. Scot-free – to write what I want to, or travel, or play, or maybe even fall in love. Boy, was I ready.

The intercom buzzed with a phone call for me. It was Dr. Figlin, my latest oncologist (Dr. Mann having moved out of state). I had phoned his office earlier to ask for the results of tests I'd taken the day before during my routine checkup. I'd had a cough for several weeks and, although it was probably a bacterial infection, we had to make sure.

"Hi, Jill. How are you?"

"You tell me, Doctor. How *am* I?"

"I'm afraid it's back."

The room spun. "The cancer?" I asked, as if he might say, "No, the Loch Ness Monster."

"Yes, Jill, the cancer. I'm so sorry."

"Does this mean I'm going to die?"

"We both know that's a possibility, Jill."

Suddenly, Dr. Barbie looked real appealing. *Come down off that screen, Dr. Barbie, and tell me this is all a bad commercial – that real life will continue in just a minute.*

Diane, my producer and friend, took me back to the office, in a state of shock, to pack up my stuff for the four months off that, fifteen minutes earlier, had seemed like a lifetime. And now . . . might be.

❧

It was a ridiculous joke that, at the very moment I was learning about the recurrence, my best friend Joni was unreachable because she was flying from her home in Chicago to mine in L.A. for a week of fun in the sun between her own chemotherapy treatments for breast cancer. It was ridiculous because four months earlier, when *she* was being diagnosed, *I* was unreachable because I was flying to meet her in Chicago, from which point we were about to depart for Spain. *Adios, España. Adios,* Fun in the Sun. And thank God Joni was on her way.

The hours between Figlin's phone call and Joni's arrival were some of the longest I'd ever numbed through. Driving to the airport, I flipped on the radio just in time to hear the song "Only the Good Die Young." For a second I thought I was living in a movie (a side effect of living in L.A.).

Speaking of movies, anyone who saw Joni and me reuniting at the airport would have sworn we were outtakes from *Beaches.* Joni – five-foot-ten, slender, stunning, with long black hair and floppy bangs covering turquoise eyes and foot-long lashes – looks and dresses like Barbara Hershey, though she sees herself as Olive Oyl. I, on the other hand, shorter and meatier, with huge red hair, have often been likened to Bette Midler. Never was I more relieved to have those spindly Olive Oyl arms around me.

Now that she'd arrived, Joni took over. She held me when I needed to be held. She listened when I needed to yell, things like "How am I gonna find a man if I'm dead?" And she joked with me when I needed to joke.

We had the weekend to somehow get through since we couldn't see Dr. Figlin and learn my options until Monday. Joni wanted to shop and eat. I wanted to clean closets and plan my estate. We compromised Saturday, and went to the movies. (*Beaches.*)

Sunday Joni persuaded me to go shopping. But my heart couldn't be in two places – my stomach and a store – at once. She'd hold up things she wanted to buy me and all I could think was *I wonder if they wear purses in Heaven; I wonder if they wear shoes in Hell.* If I were going anywhere, I wanted to pack light. Finally we settled on a pair of socks.

That night, with tears in her eyes, Joni handed over a gift she had bought me anyway, when I wasn't looking, in an antique store. A huge, unbelievably gorgeous, rose-gold pocket watch. I cried as I realized she'd bought me the one thing I could really use.

Time.

❧

When it comes to discussing cancer, especially my own, I usually hear about every tenth word. Which is why I always bring extra ears to the doctor's. On Monday, I brought Joni's, my friend Henrietta's, and my tape recorder's. And with all that listening power, I think we got about a third of the information. But here goes.

First: The cancer situation was decidedly grim. The disease appeared to have spread not only to my lungs, but to two lymph nodes in my neck. I had to face the fact that conventional medicine could no longer offer me any realistic hope of a "cure." It was time to think in terms of slowing cell growth, achieving remissions, balancing needs and hopes.

There were several options, none of them fun. I could go on hormone therapy, since there was a good chance my disease was hormonally sensitive. The hormones would not kill the cancer cells, but might "put them to rest." If I were to respond, this therapy might tide me over for one to four years, the average. When response was no longer being achieved, there would be other hormones to be tried. The side effects would be minimal, especially when compared to those of chemotherapy. It would take about three months to determine whether I was responding.

My second option was at least six months of chemotherapy. We'd know quickly if I was responding. But even if I responded beautifully, it was doubtful I could achieve a complete remission from conventional dosages. At some point I would have achieved a maximum response — the most benefit I could get from the drugs before exceeding my lifetime limit or becoming resistant to them. Then, I could go on hormone therapy in the hope of putting to rest whatever cancer cells were left. If I didn't respond to hormone therapy, there would be other chemotherapeutic regimens I could try. At that point, however, I would be on chemotherapy for the rest of my life.

After informing me of these conventional options, Dr. Figlin felt obligated to tell me about the experimental bone-marrow transplant programs that were going on at several places throughout the country. In these programs, patients were able to receive previously unthinkable doses of chemotherapy – ten to twenty-five times the conventional amounts. They were rescued from the lethal effects of such high doses by getting a transfusion of their own bone marrow, harvested and stored ahead of time. The premise was simple: The higher the amount of chemo, the higher the kill of cancer cells.

"I want *that*!" I bellowed – always a fan, when it comes to cancer, of the biggest gun I can find.

Figlin explained that to qualify for these programs you needed to have disease considered incurable by conventional treatment.

"That's *me*!" I shrieked with macabre glee. "Sign me up."

"Not so fast, Jill. You also have to show a good response to conventional treatment."

"Oh." My heart sank.

"And the transplant itself is extremely dangerous; it's not for everyone."

My soul dissolved.

"Let's talk about it after a few months, O.K.?"

I couldn't speak.

Figlin told me that, with major-organ involvement, waiting three months to see whether I'd respond to hormones was just to the left of risky. So he (and, later, another oncologist with whom he encouraged me to consult) recommended the second option – chemotherapy followed by hormone therapy. Once I calmed down, this felt right – as long as a transplant could be my reward (how weird) if I should do well on the chemo.

In the meantime, I could begin rearranging my life in all the ways made necessary by the cancer's recurrence. I would no longer be able to work regularly, but at least I wouldn't have to starve or go on the dole. During those carefree days when I was in remission, I had purchased not just medical insurance but both short-term and long-term disability insurance through my eight-month-a-year employer. Those policies now would kick in and pay my fare on the rough ride ahead.

Now that I had a plan, I actually perked up. After we left Figlin's office, Joni, Henrietta, my tape recorder and I went to my favorite restaurant for a spirited (i.e., drunken) lunch to celebrate a life-affirming decision. By then, I was so thrilled that there was something to be done that might allow me to continue this life of fried squid, caesar salad and wine, I was able to forget, for the teeniest moment, the difficult time ahead.

The day before my first chemotherapy treatment, Henrietta's husband – or as he puts it, "the best male married friend" I'll ever have – Lorenzo took me to his Chinese acupuncturist/herbalist/oncologist, Jin Lin Wang. Dr. Wang is known for his work on strengthening the immune systems of HIV-positive patients. I wanted *mine* strengthened – right away. He gave me an acupuncture treatment, accompanied by the soothing New Age tones of Kitaro. I left with a wonderfully light head and a supply of herbs. By the next morning, with four doses of herbs in me,

I felt more relaxed than I ever had on the one or two Valium I'd taken in my life.

Joni, in her own true style, surprised me by renting a white stretch limo to take me to chemotherapy. Clutching a backpack filled with "chemo toys" – relaxation and meditation tapes, a Ray Charles tape, fruit juice, hard candies, Gene Shalit's *Laughing Matters*, vomit bags and gum – I jumped into the limo, slammed Ray into the deck, lifted my arms and yelled, "Take me!" To "Unchain My Heart," Joni and I sang, danced, hugged, laughed and sobbed our way to chemo. I wanted so badly to live, if only for moments of friendship like this.

Things had changed since I'd last had chemotherapy. In 1981, before each session I'd get the shakes just anticipating the needles, nausea, vomiting and unsavory metallic taste. This time I was given a drug called Ativan to abate these side effects. But Ativan can have side effects too, one of them being short-term memory loss. People tell me I was lucid, but I remember nothing for the two days I took Ativan. Normally I hate not being in control, but this time it was a pleasure to skip it.

On the third day, when I was feeling fine, Joni regaled me with tales of my behavior – lifting the lid of my clothes hamper, thinking it was the toilet; apologizing to twenty or so perfume bottles, one at a time, after knocking them off my dresser; insisting on only one hundred percent cotton T-shirts, "no fifty-fifty!" And, not being conscious of where my bread was being buttered, criticizing cruelly Joni's shall-we-call-it cooking? "These eggs are *two* minutes, not *three*! I want *sea salt*, not Morton's! And if you want me to take my pills, you better go out and get me an apple pie from Fred Segal's!"

Meanwhile, Ativan became my drug of choice. It made chemotherapy something I didn't have to dread. Now only Joni had to.

❧

They told me I'd probably lose all my hair about two weeks after the first treatment – something that hadn't happened in my first go-round back in '81. Joni was still in town twelve days after the chemo when I received a phone call from a new man who'd gotten my number from a mutual friend. It had been forever since I'd met a new man. Or an old man. Or *any* man.

Jack was a writer who'd just moved to L.A. He was funny and clever and sensitive, it seemed, from the hour we spent just hanging out on the phone. When he finally said, "Well, let's get together," I blurted: "Yeah, I'd love to, but it's got to be right away."

Puzzled at my urgency, he asked why. I couldn't tell him, "Because my hair is scheduled to fall out in two days and I want to have just one last normal unfettered date with someone who has no idea I have cancer, before I leave for the planet Ming." So I said, "Because my sister's coming to town, day after tomorrow, and after that I might be traveling." Not *entirely* a lie.

We decided to have dinner the following night. Joni walked into the room as I was starting to describe myself so he could spot me at the restaurant (in L.A. nobody picks you up for a date). "Help me, Joni. How would you describe me?"

Loudly, so Jack could hear, she said, "Big, gorgeous honey-blonde hair and a smile that doesn't quit."

The first thing Jack said the following night was: "She was right."

Jack was adorable, exactly the kind of guy it takes me ten years to find. Attractive in kind of a quirky way, with intensely blue eyes and a terrific sense of humor. We both loved Dylan and Cocker and Paris and food. (What else is there?) We were also a match on the neurosis Richter, with commitment a word we couldn't even spell.

At the end of the evening we hugged and acknowledged we'd like to see each other again. I agreed to call him when I got "back in town."

Driving home from my last fake-normal-date-for-possibly-ever, while chuckling at something Jack had said, I started to choke. The cough that attended the cancer in my lungs yanked me off the highway, smack dab into the reality zone.

The next morning — while Joni was flying back to Chicago and I was showering and dreaming about Jack — my hair fell out in eight huge clumps.

No longer Velcroed to Joni's left hip, I filled the void of the next few days obsessing over what to do with (or with-*out*) my "big, gorgeous honey-blonde" hair. This was no small question for me — my hair had always been my one physical feature to brag on, a mainstay of my confidence out there in the critical world.

Upon my otherwise billiard-bald head remained two discreetly placed corkscrew tufts, one by each ear. They looked exactly like payess, the long sideburns worn by Hassidic Jewish men. My choices were clear: I could enter the yeshiva or buy a wig. But first, some scarves, some hats, some immediate cover, since the wig I wanted — hand-sewn, human hair – would take at least a couple of weeks.

Meanwhile, my yeshiva hair came in real handy. With those little wisps hanging out of my favorite floppy khaki hat (plus makeup, sunglasses and giant earrings) no one even knew I was bald. No one even knew I was *me*. And when those little wisps hung out of my brilliantly tied Moroccan scarf – with several deco floral-patterned scarves, time-consumingly[1] french-braided and swirled around same – strangers were literally stopping me on the street to ask how to duplicate my "statement."

It was interesting, too – my hair having always been my main feature, huge and wavy and hanging over my eyes, I'd never had to look myself square in the face. Now push had come to shove, and I had no choice. I was forced to look beyond the surface. The surprise was, the deeper I looked, the more I liked what I saw. I promised myself that if I lived long enough to grow my hair back, I'd wear it off my face and out of my eyes – though I'd never admit this to my mother.

As I write this, with my own hair – thick, rich and curlier than ever – tied back, on top of my head, I feel like I'm writing about another person. And that person amazes me. Through the whole bald boondoggle, she only cried twice. (When she put on her wig for the first time and looked like Dustin Hoffman in *Tootsie*. When some peachfuzz grew back while she was still on chemo and she was terrified it meant the drugs weren't working.)

[1] Once, late for a supper party, I explained to my hosts, "I just washed my scarves and couldn't do a thing with them."

Twice. Not that *not* crying is such a great thing. It's not. But *where was I*? Who was this person who endured the loss? What enabled her not to fold? What is that thing within us all that sustains us through nightmares we never dreamed we could bear? Is it simply the focused will to survive? Or bigger, perhaps – the willingness to LIVE? All I remember was feeling compelled to handle things with style and grace. I wanted my days, whenever they could, to burst through the half-full side of the glass, to ooze with life, drip with fun. Somehow – *some*-thank-God-*how* – the loss of my hair, the loss of my breast, the loss of control, all of these things, at the very same time, were truly horrible and no big thing. I thought . . . this is life; this is *my* life; it may not be fair; but *this is it.*

The part of me that plays to the audience helped too. She's the one who thinks about death and wonders who can be trusted to tuck her thighs into the casket just the right way, so they don't look flabby. She's the one who pictures her funeral, autumn colors, Joe Cocker blaring, Indian food and people exclaiming, "She redefined baldness . . . she answered each card . . . she clung to her payess till the very end."

Seven

❦

My response to the chemo was dramatic. After a couple of treatments my cough subsided, my breathing improved and the nodules in my neck receded. If I continued responding, I'd be investigating bone-marrow transplants after two more treatments. Since the treatments were scheduled every three weeks, this gave me a month and a half to obsess. I'd never wanted anything as badly as I wanted a transplant. Figlin encouraged me not to jump ahead, but I couldn't help it; my sights were set.

After my fourth treatment, when I was still showing a good response, Dr. Figlin arranged for me to have an interview and tests at the City of Hope hospital near Pasadena. Joni, bless that girl, came back to L.A. to accompany me. Even though she had a highly demanding job as a consultant to a quafillionaire securities broker, she'd made up her mind I'd do none of this alone. We would even turn it into a modicum of fun. The City of Hope was an hour from my home. Instead of driving back and forth for the two days of tests, we would stay at the wonderful old Huntington Hotel in Pasadena and make a little vacation out of the ordeal.

My tests included X-rays, blood work and pulmonary-function exams. The pulmonary tests terrified me – not because they were invasive or difficult; they were almost fun, blowing on these crazy machines and going inside a breathing room that looked like the contestant booth from *The $64,000 Question.* It was just that I so desperately wanted to "pass" that I became anxious, which, of course, impaired my breathing. And I was so scared they wouldn't give me a second chance if I failed. All the signs of an overachiever – I passed with flying colors.

It was the interview with the doctor that didn't go so well. To get into his program I needed not to have exceeded a certain amount of a certain chemo drug. I was devastated to learn that with my last course of treatment I had gone over the limit.

Things were getting tricky. I needed to be on conventional chemo long enough to be sure I was responding well, yet not so long that the amount of drugs I'd taken would disqualify me for a transplant. The doctor told me of another protocol for which I might qualify. This was a "phase one toxicity study." The objective seemed to be to learn how much poison a body could endure. And I would be among the first to participate.

While I was very impressed with the doctor, as well as with the City of Hope, I wanted a bigger shot at my *own* objective – to live!

❧

But time out for my birthday. On the way back from the City of Hope, Joni – who had already showered me with gifts – dragged me to one more store for one more present, a gorgeous off-white jacquard jacket with matching pants and hand-made, multi-stoned belt and earrings that took the outfit over the edge.

"This," Joni announced, as she buckled me into the belt and twirled me in front of the mirror, "is your birthday outfit." Then, sounding like a game-show hostess, she went on: "You'll be wearing it tonight to Hollywood's famous Chasen's Restaurant, favorite place of Nancy and Ronald, where I've invited twenty of your closest friends to eat our collective socks off."

When we got home, there was another surprise. Joni had flown in our mutual friend Marilyn from San Francisco. Marilyn and I had been close since high school in Detroit – Mumford, the high school Eddie Murphy put on the map when he wore a Mumford T-shirt in *Beverly Hills Cop*. We had "doubled" on my first date, my belt buckle catching on, and unraveling, Bobby Lekfowitz's sweater during Johnny Mathis's "Twelfth of Never." And on many dates after that. We were also each other's firsts – Marilyn and I – when it came to comparing sexual notes, screaming "Me-too-oh-my-Gods!" to every pent-up detail. To protect the guilty, "Crud Savage" and "Harvey Fingers" were the code names we gave the first boys who ever touched our breasts. In 1982, just six months after me, Marilyn was diagnosed with breast cancer.

And now . . . here we were, the three girlfriends, all with breast cancer, squashed into my bathroom, bopping and dressing to the Pointer Sisters, a slow-motion version of the deodorant commercial where the nineteen-year-olds get gorgeous in thirty seconds for their dates. *Real* slow-motion. With two wigs (Joni's and mine), two prostheses (Mar's and mine), one hip brace (Joni's from an unrelated disorder), and six shoulderpads (the only things *all* of us had), we needed the disclaimer "Some Assembly Required." It was Marilyn who, noticing how funny we looked with four breasts among the three of us, screamed: "I know . . . we'll call ourselves 'The Pointless Sisters!'"

The evening was magical. Our table was perfect – oval, so people weren't too far apart, in a semi-private area of the restaurant by leaded-glass windows with a garden view. I sat there a while just looking around, scanning the faces, reviewing my life, playing games with myself, like how many people had I known during my marriage, how many came after, how many before?

I laughed as I tallied the stats on the men. There were two Davids. One was my first date in high school in 1959 (I wore a shiny navy-blue sheath from J.L. Hudson's and my first two-inch heels from Chandler's). The other was my first date after my marriage ended in 1983 (I wore jeans, a peach T-shirt and a hippy-dippy jacket of way too many colors).

Then there were the Michaels. Three of them: The Michael I loved but never slept with. The Michael I slept with but never loved. And the Michael I wrote songs with, never slept with and *could* have loved, but when *I* was married, *he* wasn't, and when *I* wasn't, *he* was. There's a snapshot from that evening of me, *that* Michael and his wife – well, actually she's mostly out of frame, so all you see of *her* is a smidgen of her head, which is resting in her hand, which is covering her eye, which is lucky for us all, because if she could've seen the way Michael and I were looking at each other, the evening might've taken an ugly turn.

Meanwhile, everyone brought me hysterical gifts and

ridiculously wonderful poems and cards – all of which showed me how truly they knew me, how dearly they cared, how deeply they'd miss me . . .

The unspoken thought that it might be my last pushed this birthday right to the wall. Even our waiter sensed something was up. At the end of the evening he gave me a hug and said, "Never have I seen a celebration so rich with passion, so filled with life."

The next day, I called M.D. Anderson Cancer Center in Houston. From preliminary phone conversations, the program there appealed to me and it sounded like I might be an excellent candidate. Timing was critical, however. I needed to be there the following day for two days of tests and, if I qualified, be ready to enter the program immediately. If I didn't qualify, I needed to be back in L.A. within a few days in order not to interrupt my conventional treatment. With head-spinning speed, I collected my medical records from all over the city and packed and closed up business as if I were going to be gone for over three months. That's how long the procedure would take.

Meanwhile, Joni turned on a dime, canceling her next few days of appointments in Chicago so she could join me in Houston, keeping her promise – I'd do none of this alone.

The first day, Thursday, was wonderful. I loved the doctor. I loved the program. I loved the hospital. *I loved life.* I had blood tests and a CAT scan of the chest. Then they scheduled my bone-marrow harvest for the next Tuesday, to be followed by chemotherapy and the transplant, assuming all went well with an initial marrow biopsy scheduled for the morning after my arrival.

That evening, we ordered room service, took bubble baths, drank champagne and called all my friends to tell them the good news — I'd been scheduled for the transplant; this must mean I was an excellent candidate, since I'd always assumed research doctors don't like to screw up their numbers by accepting poor risks.

If you're ever in the market for a bone-marrow biopsy, Anderson's the place. All my fears about the procedure were dispelled the next day by two extremely gentle nurses. Wanting to spare Joni, who is certifiably needle-phobic, I asked her to wait outside as the nurses put me on a table, butt side up. They began to give me shots to numb the area around my hips. Suddenly, something that felt like a fish plopped into my hand. I looked up to discover a disgustingly clammy Joni who'd returned to transcend her phobia in the ultimate act of friendship. I pressed my forehead into hers, shielding her from the sight, as the nurses began to drill for my marrow.

"It's not that . . . ouch . . . bad, Joni. Really, it's not. Joni? Joni? Oy! Joni? Are you O.K.? I can't feel a . . . oh, my God . . . no, no, Joni, just kidding, it tickles. Joni? Oh, Joni-i-i-? Check on her, gentle nurses. Please!"

I was so busy protecting the most precious friend I could ever have, the whole thing was over before I knew it.

And now, once again, Joni and I had a weekend of waiting to get through. But not to worry; our calendar was full. The main event would be the writing of my will. Having no children, no husband, and, more importantly, no assets, I'd never written one, but now, with a fifteen percent chance of dying from the transplant, it seemed like the thing to do. By Sunday evening I'd left all of my earthly writings to Joni, my Grateful Dead records and T-shirts to my nephews, my peach hooded robe to my sister Carol, my army jacket with the propeller buttons to my sister Mindy, and my entire chemotherapy hat collection to the best *bald* male married friend I'll ever have, Lorenzo. Clearly the will of a twelve-year-old.

I awoke Monday morning excited and hopeful. We could start the ball rolling, or as my dad always said, get the show on the road. I phoned the hospital to find out the results of my bone-marrow biopsy, but my doctor had been called out of town for the day. He would see me on Tuesday morning, before my harvest.

In the afternoon, I called again and somehow persuaded the nurse to disclose the biopsy results over the phone. I'll never stop hearing her monotonal Texas drawl as she read to me, "Left side, no evidence of metastatic breast cancer. Right side, *evidence* of metastatic breast cancer." I was sure I'd heard wrong. It just couldn't be. None of my doctors thought the cancer would actually be in my marrow. Now that it was found there, however, the harvest was canceled; I couldn't have the transplant.

I've never been lower than I was in that moment. In one little sentence, all my dreams had been shattered. I was no longer eligible for the only procedure that offered me any hope of seeing my two-year-old niece grow up. My spirits had been so high; now I needed to be scraped off the floor.

Henrietta phoned that evening. When she heard the news and, more importantly, my tone, she firmly announced, "I'll be there tomorrow." Since Joni had to leave the next morning, and since the thought of flying back to L.A. alone felt like throwing a funeral and having no one show up, I didn't argue; I just took a deep breath and sobbed goodbye.

About a year earlier – when I'd been having horrible headaches and was afraid the cancer had spread to my brain – it was Henrietta who invited me, on behalf of Lorenzo and herself, to die in their home if it ever came to that. I was thoroughly touched, totally relieved. I also felt guilty, so I promised her that if it ever *did* come to that, I'd make sure we had fun. Later, I called Lorenzo to thank him for the invite.

"Hi," he said, cheerfully. "I hear you have a brain tumor."

"Not any more. My headache's gone. But thanks for inviting me to live with you."

Knowing how to handle me, as always, he shot back: "We didn't say *live.*"

❧

Tuesday, with tag-team precision, Henrietta arrived as Joni was leaving, the two of them quickly hugging hello and goodbye at high noon in the clinic reception room where Joni and I had been waiting three hours for my alleged morning appointment. In fairness, the doctor *had* popped into the waiting area briefly to apologize for being late and assure me that we just had to get rid of a "few little cells" and then we'd be back on track. I had no idea what he meant, but I allowed his casually confident air to pull me back down to earth. Or, at least, earth as I'd come to know it – that special place where my only tasks were to eat, sleep, excrete, breathe and not think more than a millisecond ahead.

Our appointment, when we finally had it, actually gave

me back some hope. While it was true I couldn't proceed with the transplant then, the doctor said that if my marrow were to clear after some more conventional chemo, I might be eligible later on. There was also something else I should investigate right away, he said. It was called a peripheral stem-cell transplant.

Stem cells, which circulate in the blood, perform the same function as bone marrow: They produce infection-fighting white blood cells. And even in a case like mine, when the bone marrow is contaminated with cancer, there's a good chance that the stem cells aren't. So a transplant procedure had been devised for them, too. Like bone marrow, the stem cells would have to be harvested from my body – but not in a surgical procedure under general anesthesia, as with the marrow. Instead, stem cells are gathered by drawing the blood into a machine that culls them out and then returns the blood to the patient. But the rest of the procedure would be the same – high-dose chemotherapy followed by stem-cell or bone-marrow transfusion and a vulnerable wait for the white cells to engraft and resume their function.

My doctor in Houston recommended a Dr. William Vaughan, who at that time was at the University of Nebraska Medical Center and was running a peripheral stem-cell transplant program for breast cancer. I would go back to L.A., have a few more treatments of conventional chemotherapy and, sometime in between them, go to Nebraska to check out his program.

As devastated as I was that the cancer had spread farther than originally suspected –tests in Houston also revealed metastases in my spine and ribs – I left feeling less flattened than I had. My window of opportunity had not completely closed. There was still something left to do. Grateful, and in serious need of celebration, Henrietta and I invited the doctor to dinner, where wine, pasta and lots of jokes created a temporary state of grace.

A few hours later, we left for L.A. on the "red-eye" in order to make my morning appointment for the conventional chemo I had been hoping not to resume. By then, I had sobered into the horror of what I was facing and had absolutely no inkling of where I would find the strength to regroup.

Eight

❦

Usually, I bopped into chemo wearing my "Young Hearts '88 – Head Over Heels" T-shirt, sweats and an over-compensatory smile, blathering endlessly about God knows what, trying with all my might to turn a nightmare into a circus. This time I was silent.

Susan, my chemo nurse, asked me if Dr. Figlin had changed my drugs now that they'd found the cancer in new places. That, too, hit me hard. It had been one thing not to be able to have the transplant. But now for the first time it dawned on me that my prognosis might have worsened. (*Worsened*? What's the difference between dead and very dead?)

As it turned out, my drugs stayed the same. And another new fear – that the cancer had been growing while I was on chemo – receded, too. More likely, the "new" sites had been there right along; we just hadn't tested for them. Furthermore, who was to say there hadn't been *more* cancer in my bones and marrow *before* I started the chemo? With no baseline for those sites, I could assume I was getting better.

This quasi-positive thinking held me for at least ten minutes until the Ativan began to course through my veins and take me to that special place where thinking isn't a problem.

But two days later, when I returned to the planet, I was certifiably depressed. And then certifiably *obsessed.* Having decided to write the doctor in Houston and thank him for his care, I must've written the note twenty-five times. Several times I changed how I wrote the letter "E" (sometimes so it looked like a backward "3," other times like a normal "E," but always so *every* "E" in the note was the same; and if I blew it, I threw the whole note out). After I got my cursive under control, I began to perseverate over punctuation, back and forth, forth and back, until my head felt like a lighthouse. Finally – when I'd written the note so many times that it no longer made sense to me – I began to change words.

The most pathetic part, though, was that every time I changed punctuation and every time I changed a word, I called Joni in Chicago to run it past her. It's no exaggeration to say that, in regard to a little five-sentence note, I called Joni at least twenty times. The first nineteen times she was extremely patient, the gentleness in her voice a clue that she knew she was dealing with a psycho. On the twentieth call, regarding whether to put an exclamation point after "Great dinner," she very calmly said, "Jill-l-l," then screamed, "MAIL IT!!!!!"

I hung up and wrote the note several more times, knowing what Joni couldn't possibly know – that the perfect note was the *only* thing that could save my life.

❧

I later learned that much of my depression, as well as my obsession, was chemically based. One of the anti-side-effect drugs I'd been taking had its *own* side effect of making every millisecond seem like a year – an excruciating experience when all I was trying to do was get through each day. Once I learned this, I understood why Selma Checkonowsky's chicken sandwich had sent me to the planet Pluto.

Selma, my wonderful across-the-hall neighbor, was somewhere in her late eighties. Four feet tall and fragile, yet very independent, she moved in slow motion in *real* life and wouldn't allow anyone to help her. The day I was writing the perfect note, she shuffled by and invited me over for a chicken sandwich. I told her I'd be there as soon as I finished my note. Two hours later, I knocked on her door.

Tiny footsteps. Little clunkettes. Slowly. Slowly. Oh-dear-Lord-please-hurry-up. Selma's fumbling to open the door seemed to last from winter to spring.

As I entered, she asked me to wait; she wanted to "run" down and pick up the mail. Uh-oh. Two flights of stairs. Round trip. Real time or drug time, it didn't matter; a voice inside me silently screamed. I offered . . . begged . . . to do it for her. But she refused.

A millennium later, I followed her to the kitchen table, where the smallest chicken I'd ever seen grew to turkey proportion in relation to Selma. At a pace that would make a snail look like thunder, she meticulously severed a thigh, removed the skin, placed the meat on a cutting board, trekked all-l-l the way-y-y-y across the kitchen, opened a drawer, took out some Saran Wrap, trekked all-l-l the way-y-y-y back to the table and there wrestled slowly with the Saran Wrap until the remainder of Mr. Chicken was hermetically sealed.

After that, Selma set sail, again, for the other side of the kitchen, to return the Saran Wrap – I don't know – before it got stale?

I could no longer bear it. In counterpoint to the rest of my world standing painfully still, my heart and soul began to race. My hands were trembling. My face was on fire, and my eyes were twirling out of their sockets. When Selma finally lifted her weapon, to carve, and said, "I like mine *real* thin, how about you?" – I grabbed the thigh and screamed:

"I like mine *whole*!"

When I went for my next oncology checkup, my white blood count had taken a dive.

"If you were scheduled for chemo today, we'd have to cancel," Figlin told me. "But you still have a week, so let's see what happens."

On the way out, I stopped to chat with some of my nurse friends and franti-casually queried, "How can I bring my blood count up?"

"Red meat," they answered in unison.

That weekend I was going to San Francisco to meet Joni and some friends for several large meals. Determined to bring my count up, I pledged to eat red meat (something I hadn't done in seventeen years) every chance I got. What I really wanted, if I were going to do this, was a "Double Cheese Whopper, extra pickles, cut." But at Friday night's restaurant I had to settle for a sixteen-ounce porterhouse steak.

Then at 4 in the morning I woke Joni and said to her, in the language of best friends, "Room service-ez-vous?" Her face lit up. She grabbed the phone.

"I'll have a cheeseburger," I said, Groucho-ing my brows and adding, "for medicinal purposes, of course."

Said Joni: "I hate to see you eat red meat alone."

I had a cheese-mushroom-bacon-onion-pickle-burger with cremated fries and a chocolate shake. Joni had steak, eggs, sausage, butter-drenched toast and real coffee – foods that hadn't touched her lips for a minimum of fourteen years.

For lunch and dinner we had giant steaks. And for late-afternoon snacks, room-service chili.

The following day, for variety's sake, we had lamb chops for breakfast, burgers for lunch, steaks for snacks. And barf bags for dinner. Joni spent the evening in the bathroom. I spent it with a fender in my stomach, afraid to bend, afraid to move.

It all seemed worth it the following week when my white blood count had jumped back up.

"It worked," I announced to Dr. Figlin.

"What worked?"

"Well, last week I asked the nurses how I could help my count and they said red meat, so I've eaten nothing but cow for an entire week."

"Too bad," he said.

"Why?"

"You should've been more specific when you asked the nurses. Red meat only helps your *red* blood count."

"Not my white?"

"That's right."

I ran to the bathroom and threw up my breakfast. A Double Cheese Whopper, extra pickles, cut.

To avoid the disappointment I'd experienced in Houston, I left for Omaha maintaining the attitude that I was casually going to check out the stem-cell transplant program and, if it seemed plausible, I'd consider it an option. That didn't work, of course. By the time I arrived in Omaha, I was certain the cancer was growing in my lungs – on the plane I developed a cough; in the airport I developed emphysema. In the cab I developed heart failure; I have never felt so anxious. I tried to calm down with a meditation tape. A soothing voice told me to picture the word "relax," but I kept seeing it backward – "xaler." Now, along with everything else, I had to wonder: Had I suddenly become dyslexic or had the tumor merely spread to my brain?

Joni, of course, met me in Omaha and took over breathing for me. Though we'd sworn off the stuff, we treated ourselves to a steak dinner, figuring when in Rome . . .

The next morning we met with the transplant coordinator and Dr. Vaughan. Looking at my records, they thought I'd be a "decent" candidate, pending final testing. They explained the risks – respiratory failure, kidney failure, heart failure, bleeding, infection, and so on. They explained the major benefit – a chance at life or, at least, a longer disease- and chemo-free interval than achievable with conventional treatment. The number of people who had gone through this procedure anywhere was small; the number who'd gone through the program in Omaha was fewer than twenty. But, based on these small numbers, the statistics were: A sixty percent chance of responding to the treatment and achieving complete remission. For those who responded, a fifty percent chance of relapsing within the first year. For those who didn't relapse in the first year, a fifty percent chance of relapsing in the second year. Nobody had been "out" long enough to project farther ahead than that. But there seemed to be some promising results.

The bottom line was – a big risk for a little shot at a possible long-term gain. As big as the risk, as little as the shot, it still offered me more than conventional treatment. I wanted it.

Dr. Vaughan felt that, if final testing showed I was a candidate, the moment to begin the procedure was upon us; any more conventional chemotherapy could compromise my bone marrow too much for a transplant. He scheduled me for a brain scan, the first of several crucial tests. If I had brain metastases I would be ineligible. It would be curtains. That would be that. During the scan I tried to relax, but all I could see was "x-a-l-e-r, x-a-l-e-r."

The results of my brain scan would not be available for twenty-four hours – which was long enough for another emotional roller coaster to get going. Back at the hotel I phoned my doctor in Houston to discuss the events of the day. I told him about Dr. Vaughan's feeling that I should have the stem-cell transplant now – and was shocked to discover that he disagreed. His reasons were complex: He still wanted to see if my bone marrow would clear with a few more courses of conventional therapy. If it did, he said, he could put me back in his transplant program, which offered stronger chemotherapy than the one in Omaha. Furthermore, he said, if my marrow *didn't* clear with conventional treatment, that probably would mean that *neither* type of transplant program offered much hope – in other words, if I understood him correctly, I might as well wait; there was nothing to lose.

In that moment, my heart sank to a place from which it's never returned.

To confuse matters more, the Texas doctor went on to say that maybe I could have a stem-cell transplant, later on, with him. Did he have a program up and running? Not yet. So what was he offering? Advice, I guess. And well-intentioned. But advice that knocked the wind from my sails. I was thoroughly confused, and so shocked I couldn't speak with him further.

After we hung up, I was reeling with questions. What if I continued conventional treatment and my bone marrow didn't clear? Would I feel that a stem-cell transplant was better than nothing at all? Probably. And, if so, *and* if there wasn't a program up and running in Houston, would I still be eligible for the Omaha program? Even if my bone marrow *did* clear, might it by then be too compromised for a transplant? Or worse, could a clear biopsy be a sampling error? Imagine going to all the trouble of a transplant only to give myself back my own cancer. (Several doctors told me this was certainly a possibility.) And, cleared marrow or not, what if my general condition worsened in the months I stayed on conventional treatment? Would I still be strong enough to endure a transplant? Would I still be eligible for *any* program? And let's say my bone marrow *didn't* clear and I decided to have a stem-cell transplant – would I be able to wipe out the thought he'd planted that it probably wouldn't really help? Would I ever be able to recapture the original faith I'd invested in the procedure – the faith that made me want it more than anything, and also gave me the strength to stand it?

My head was spinning. I had thought I was just waiting to see if I had brain metastases. Now, if my brain was O.K., I had to use it *real hard* to decide between the conflicting advice of two fine doctors; both of whom I respected; both of whom I believed.

I tried to put it all aside till the next day, when I'd know about my brain scan. But there was no way. Every fifteen minutes I completely changed my mind about what to do.

After hours of this, I announced to Joni, "I feel like a schizophrenic."

"Don't worry," she said, without skipping a beat. "Tomorrow you'll feel like another person."

It's amazing what makes you jump up and down and shout "hallelujah" once you're traveling the cancer road. My brain scan was normal. Oh, what a feeling!

By now it was Friday. Dr. Vaughan said that, if I decided to enter his program, we could start collecting stem cells the following Wednesday. I was scheduled for my next conventional chemotherapy treatment back in L.A. the following Thursday. This meant I had four days to make my decision.

My first decision was *not* to go home. Instead, I would spend a long weekend in Denver, where my sister Mindy lived with her husband, Art, and their daughter, Gracie. Family was what I needed – especially the innocence of my two-year-old niece. I was praying for those moments of richness and purity that you can only have with a child. Instead, I experienced the worst four days of my life.

From the minute I landed, I was on the phone, hashing and rehashing my complicated options – with my therapist in L.A., with my friends across the country, and with every oncologist I'd ever known. When I wasn't on the phone I was waiting for doctors to return my calls, so I wouldn't leave the house even for a minute. I became so anxious about missing one call while taking another that my sister sweet-talked the phone company into installing "immediate emergency call-waiting."

After three days of this I sent Mindy to the store for an answering machine so we could go out to dinner and not miss a call. Then I spent the whole evening on the restaurant phone, calling the machine to see if I'd missed a call. *Help*!

My therapist, Penelope, was wonderful. Over the phone, she helped me regulate my breathing. She also taught me how to meditate. Talk about listening to the sounds of silence.

The doctors I consulted were incredible too. Each one made himself or herself available over a weekend and, in three cases, while they were out of town at the same convention. Dr. Figlin was more than willing to set up a conference call with Joni and me at 7 in the morning from a hotel where he was vacationing. "How long do we have?" I asked him. He answered, "As long as it takes."

I asked thousands of questions and took tons of notes. Things would get clear and then I would lose it. By the end of the weekend I was thoroughly confused. But I kept on going. I'd make notes on my notes, add questions to my questions and call whomever I needed for answers. I was trying to gather all the information I possibly could on something about which little was known. One second I would think to myself, if I have a stem-cell transplant now, I'll never know for sure if my marrow would've cleared on conventional treatment. Then I would think, well, I can always assume that it *would've* cleared and, therefore, recapture the belief and spirit I desperately need in order to endure the transplant. The next second, my thinking would flip to . . . but what if my marrow was never going to clear? Will I be putting myself through a futile process? Or if it *was* going to clear, will I be giving myself less chemo than would be effective, if only I could be patient enough to wait a few months to see if I'm eligible for the Houston program? But what's enough chemo, anyway? If Omaha's is three-fourths of Houston's, who's to say that isn't enough? Why would they bother to design a program with *not enough*?

I was going nuts. Coughing, forgetting to breathe, churning, obsessing, and never – despite incredible support – feeling more desperate or more alone. It finally became clear, though, that I had to base my decision on what was available to me *then* – at that exact moment in my cancer life – not on something months down the line that didn't now exist, and might never, in Houston. So I was zeroing in, but still not quite home.

Since no oncologist (except for the Texan) was willing to make a flat recommendation, I tried the old question "If it were you, what would you do?" Or "If it were your wife – *and you loved her* – what would you hope *she* would do?" One doctor, a woman, admitted she'd go for the stem-cell transplant. Another doctor admitted he'd want his wife to investigate the procedure, but wasn't ready to say what he'd want her to do. Another was willing to tell a friend of mine – but not me, directly – that, while he had trouble picturing his wife doing it, he really thought *I* should. The shocker came when I asked my favorite doctor, one of the few who had been guiding me down the transplant path, and he said, basically, that he would *not* want his wife to endure a transplant; he'd rather have her home for however long she had.

Strangely enough, it was hearing *this*, together with two other things I learned, that enabled me to squeeze my decision out of the turnip. First, I learned that a transplant with high-dose chemotherapy could make me resistant to further chemo, should I need it down the line. Second, I learned that if I survived the transplant, but the chemo failed, my life would probably be shorter than if I stayed on conventional chemotherapy. Or as one doctor put it, "If you want to be alive ten years from now, have the transplant. If you want to be alive one year from now, don't."

Now that I understood the bleakest possible scenario, I was able to put down my notes, get quiet and wait for an answer to come from somewhere deep inside. In my evening meditation, with my breathing even, with my heart and mind calm, these words came:

"*Even if it's shorter, the quality of my life will be better because what living I do will be done knowing I'd given it my best shot.*"

And with that, I jumped up, ran to my niece and cried, "C'mon, Gracie, we're taking a bath!"

We threw off our clothes, hopped in the tub, splashed, dunked, squealed, giggled, and, two hours later, emerged — shriveled, radiant, and thoroughly cleansed.

Nine

❦

The evening after I made my decision, Mindy and Gracie flew back with me to Omaha. My parents, bless their hearts, had already flown in from Detroit and scoured the city to find us the only available places to stay: Two apartments, one for them and one for me and whomever was visiting, much like the apartments I'd lived in as a college student in the sixties. The smell of cigarettes wrapped in steak fat permeated the halls. Having a transplant started to take on the odor of final exams.

That evening, Joni called to tell me her phone was ringing off the hook with people who wanted to come be with me. She'd already whipped out her neurotic little crocodile Filofax and carefully scheduled several weeks of nonstop, non-overlap, perfectly timed, and perfectly appropriate visitors. My folks would stay with me through the entire ordeal, but now they would also have some relief. I was overwhelmed by the outpouring of love and support that had only just begun.

The next day, Mindy and I went to the outpatient clinic to begin collecting my blood for the stem-cell harvest. There I met my blood brother, Dryden (an Army officer who'd left his base to join the Army of Life – his battle, non-Hodgkin's lymphoma), and my blood sister, Melissa (an inside-out gorgeous twenty-year-old college student, also battling non-Hodgkin's lymphoma). The three of us would be together for as long as it took us to get the stem cells we each needed. The procedure was called pheresis *(fah-rē ces)* and the room was the pheresis room, so I decided we all must be a bunch of pheresis monkeys. As in any war, Dryden, Melissa, and I were best friends within twenty seconds.

The process is not painful. It's like having an I.V. We would each be hooked up to a pheresis machine for the same four hours every day. During that time we would undergo as many "cycles" of blood as we could. A cycle would consist of the machine's drawing our blood, spinning it to separate out the stem cells, then giving back the remaining blood. The speed at which each of us could tolerate this would vary and, therefore, so would the total number of cycles per day. With no premeditation, without even a hint at an oral agreement, we all began the Stem-Cell Olympics, secretly peering at each other's "scores," not so much wanting to beat each other as definitely not wanting to lag behind. A score of nine to twelve cycles per day was considered a victory.

It was determined on the first day that Melissa's and my veins would not be able to withstand pheresis. This wasn't uncommon, but it meant we had to have a catheter, or hollow tube, surgically inserted into our veins through which to collect our blood. Dryden's veins were fine, of course. Now we were talking the boys versus the girls!

The surgery was a piece of cake. Local anesthesia; I hardly felt a thing. In the recovery room, however, a nurse eventually asked me, "Are you strong enough to walk?" When I told her not yet, she whined, "Aw, c'mon, give it a try." So I said, "O.K., but first please help me to the bathroom." She dragged me there, I entered, and, quite by habit, locked myself in. The next thing I remember was someone banging on the door while I muttered, "I'm finding myself on the floor here." I did manage to open the door and walk out; not long after that, I woke up in an oxygen tent with a gash on my head. Apparently I had fainted and fallen twice. My surgeon was there checking me out while the nurse who'd originally questioned me was defending herself with "But she told me she was ready to walk!" If this was the quality of care awaiting me, she was right – I *was* ready to walk.

As it turned out, that particular nurse was an aberration. The other good news – the girls won! Our catheters seemed to enable more cycles per day than Dryden's macho veins. After six days, I'd collected enough stem cells. I think it took Dryden over two weeks.

Catheter in place, Valium in hand, my next job was to endure several more days of tests to make sure the cancer hadn't spread since Houston. At this point the thought that anything could possibly keep me from moving forward was more than I could bear. Fortunately, Dale and Steffie, my friends since high school, had arrived to spend five glorious days holding my increasingly sweaty hands. Their lives, unfortunately, had prepared them for this moment. Dale, a diabetic since childhood, had undergone two heart bypass surgeries before the age of forty. And Steffie is my friend whose daughter – thanks to experimental laser surgery – had survived a brain tumor three years prior. So no one here was a stranger to living on the edge.

We got through the time between tests picnicking on junk food in the ugly park across from my apartment and playing Boggle, that game where you form as many words as you can with a bunch of lettered dice. How come I kept finding words like "nurse," "doctor," "needles," and "vomit"? On the last day of Steffie and Dale's visit, Joni flew in for the meeting with the doctor in which we would find out if I was truly, totally in the program. While we waited for him in the examining room, the three of them kept reminding me to breathe.

When Dr. Vaughan finally arrived, it was only to tell us the results of my tests had been delayed until the afternoon. He also told us he'd just learned that my insurance company had denied me coverage on the basis that transplants for breast cancer were still experimental. This meant that, even if all the tests came back fine, I couldn't be admitted to the hospital without a letter of credit for $120,000 (80 percent of the estimated cost). Well! At least we had something to divert us while we awaited the test results.

At lunch I told the story I'd recently heard of a man who sued his insurance company because it wouldn't cover his bone-marrow transplant. He won the case, but it took six months. The problem was, by then he was dead.

We immediately started mental fund-raising. Steffie offered to sell a painting that hung in her dining room. She figured it could get us $15,000. Joni was good for several thousand. Dale had a bundle in shoeboxes under her bed. And I just happened to have a box of 500 unused Mumford High School pencils. Now that the school was a movie star, there was no telling what those could fetch.

The more we talked, the more ridiculous it got. If I passed my final tests, I needed to be admitted the following Monday. It was already Friday. How were we going to raise $120,000 in two short days? There was nothing left to do but eat chocolate chip cookies and Junior Mints until 3:00, when we'd return to the doctor.

By then the results were in. I passed my tests. Yahoo. But now what? Every inch of this journey was leaving me breathless.

There is no word but "miracle" for what happened minutes later. While we were talking with Dr. Vaughan about the Catch-22 of it all, a nurse knocked on his door to call me to the phone. I excused myself, extremely puzzled. Who would be seeking me out here at the clinic?

It was my father calling to tell me that the man for whom he'd worked for the last 50 years had offered us the $120,000.

I found out later that only a few days earlier this man's son had died. I don't know exactly what that event had to do with his generosity, but it made receiving it all the more meaningful.

What came my way next in terms of support was a relay race of the heart – a chain of friends who would literally hug as they'd pass each other in the Omaha airport. In the first heat, Steffie, Dale and Joni left as Harriet arrived from Montreal, where she'd moved. And Harriet, most compulsive of all my friends, was perfectly suited for the task ahead, a weekend of bill-paying, bank-balancing, file-making, and dread.

On Monday morning, my mother, my father and Harriet checked me into the University of Nebraska Medical Center or, as I liked to call it, the Transplant Hilton. Though in some numb corner of my frazzled brain I must've been scared, the relief of having gotten past all the decision-making, cancer testing, and money issues transformed my terror into blissful surrender.

Before I was taken up to my room, Harriet and I slipped away, protecting my parents from my second-to-last piece of civilian business – the signing of my will. It was witnessed by Harriet, God and my two closest friends – a nurse and receptionist I'd never met before and would never meet again.

The door of my room had been decorated by some nurses. Amid a lush background of greenery was a sign that read "Jill's Jungle." At my Rousseau door, I performed the ritual of all those who would ever enter: the washing of the hands; the donning of the gown; and then, upon entering, one more washing of the hands. Having entered the world of "modified protective isolation," it was weird to realize, when the door closed behind me, that I would not leave this room for at least six weeks. Fortunately, they gave me a room with a view. Unfortunately, the view was a cemetery.

❧

Joni would be returning to Omaha that evening. Knowing how passionate she was about decorating, I immediately angled my hospital bed and Barcalounger chairs.

And lucky I did. At 6:00 sharp, my fanatic fairy-godmother friend twirled through the door with a fleet of peach and seafoam-green decorating items – pillows, comforters, throws, rugs, lamps, paintings, picture frames, jars – and whipped that place into such amazing shape that within minutes I was praying my room would go condo.

We sent out for wine and an elaborate Indian dinner – the last solid food I would have for four weeks. Then, while we waited for it to arrive, we set about finishing my *last* little bit of real-life business. It was time to adhere to the Jewish tradition whereby someone who is very ill changes his or her name to fool the Angel of Death. I had entered the hospital as Jill. I would leave the hospital as someone else. And tonight we would figure out who.

I closed my eyes and got real quiet, employing the new meditation skills Penelope had taught me over the phone. And they worked. Within seconds I *saw* my new name – Fanny. Fanny! It surprised *me* as much as it did everyone else.

"Is Fanny a name you're sure you can live with?" my mother asked.

"I hope so, Mother. God, I hope so."

Afraid of messing up my medical records, I never told the hospital staff I'd decided to change my name. Besides, choosing a new name was one thing, using it quite another. I wasn't ready; I wasn't sure why. But somehow I needed to let it be Jill who endured the uncertainty of the weeks ahead.

The morning after my "Last Supper," I was scheduled

for a bronchoscopy. That's where they stick a scope down your throat and into your lungs to see what's going on, the lungs being one of the more vulnerable places for serious infection during transplant. A nurse was thoughtless enough to tell me that a lot of people said a bronchoscopy felt like drowning. That gave me something to look forward to.

Harriet was with me when the bronchoscopy team arrived – two funny and sympathetic people, a nurse named Jane and a doctor named Joe. They said I could use my Walkman during the procedure. So with Valium, a fabulous job of throat-numbing (thank you, Jane) and relaxation tapes dulceting through my earphones, I didn't even gag as they carefully guided what felt like a garden hose down my throat and into my lungs. For the record, a bronchoscopy is *not* like drowning and that nurse should be shot.

That afternoon, I went back to the catheter folks to have another couple of "lines" put in. The first catheter, for pheresis, had been inserted because my veins were lousy. Now I needed more lines to help ward off infection once the heavy-duty chemo started. It would kill off my white blood cells, and then I wouldn't be able to have any shots because the needles could cause infection. So any medication I needed would have to come through a catheter. I would keep my first one, which exited from my right side, just below my waist. The new lines would exit from my chest and hang there like elongated Frederick's of Hollywood pasties.

Harriet joined me for the surgery. We chatted through much of it, distancing ourselves from the actual event by watching it on a monitor; it was happening to the TV, not me.

When we returned to my room, we were greeted by

Florence Frightingale – the one who'd warned me that a bronchoscopy was like drowning. As she tucked me into bed, she told me all about a man who bent down one day, stepped on the end of his catheter without realizing it, then stood up and yanked the whole thing out of his chest.

I thanked her for sharing.

❧

There was no rest for the wicked at the Transplant Hilton. Hours after the bronchoscopy and catheter surgery, I began my week of high-dose chemotherapy. Joni, Harriet, my parents, and my sister Carol were with me, in round-the-clock shifts, through every minute, their love and devotion an antidote to each deadly drop of mystery elixir that journeyed through my veins.

And, boy, my veins were really hopping. Figuratively and literally, I was wired – connected to an I.V. pole I named Ivan. Ivan had a body made of square metal monitors, one for his chest and one for his stomach – a robot's stomach, with numbers that went up as my medicine went down. And Ivan, you might say, became my main man. He nourished me – with something called TPN for total nutrition, with antibiotics to prevent infection, and with my chemo and side-effects drugs. Our song, a computerized rendition of Beethoven's Fifth, would blare from his tin heart whenever my I.V. bags were on empty. We went everywhere together, Ivan and me. Which was mostly to the bathroom.

Beyond that, what I'm able to recall of my week of chemo you can put in a thimble, since once again I took Ativan, my short-term-memory-loss drug of choice. I'm told, however, that every day I telephoned friends and, while I wasn't exactly Chatty Cathy, I certainly held my own. It also appears I was very demanding when it came to fashion – always giving color preferences for hospital gowns, with two back-up choices in case they were out of my favorites, "the green ones with all the little circles, each one about a centimeter apart from the next." Strangely enough, I *do* remember *one* thing – showering every morning and thinking, "This chemo's not that bad."

After seven days of chemo I had a "day of rest" and a changing of the guard. Joni and Harriet left as Judith, a friend since the sixties, arrived. Judith, an artist, oozes life. She was currently working on a painting in my honor, pouring healing energy into her canvas, and out to me, from the deepest place she knew.

The transplant took place the next day. My stem cells had been collected in nine bags. Now, Judith and my family watched as a nurse named Kim took the first of those bags out of a freezer and laid it in a warm pan of water to thaw – a ritual bath. As soon as it thawed, Kim rushed it over, hung it on Ivan, hooked it up to one of my catheters and announced, "Bag one." This went on for several hours, one transfusion after another, until finally Kim announced, "Bag nine!" All the while I'd been in and out of awareness, due to sedation, but always awake for the counting of the bags.

When I heard "bag nine," I looked over at Judith – and started to laugh. Her appearance had altered strangely. She was still wearing the requisite yellow mid-calf isolation gown, but hanging out from under it, instead of the white slacks she'd worn earlier, was a pair of my favorite hospital jammies, the green ones with the little circles about a centimeter apart. When I asked her why, she said: "You're not going to believe this, but the minute your first bag of blood started dripping, so did *I*." Judith had gotten her period – two weeks early. What a friend.

With the ninth bag completed, Judith, an expert in numerology, told me the significance of the number nine. It's the end of a cycle, the beginning of something new. The moment she said it, it all made sense – the chemo had been the end of Jill; the transplant, the beginning of Fanny. Like the sacrificial lamb, Jill had to die so Fanny could live.

Judith had to leave Omaha the morning after the transplant. When she came to the hospital to say goodbye, she was shocked to find me riding and singing on the exercise bike in my room to *The Phantom of the Opera's* "Music of the Night." I hadn't felt this alive since surviving a near-fatal scuba dive in 1975.

Judith was carrying a gift. Ironically, it was a beautiful two-piece sculpture of a woman doing a handstand on a bike. Now I wanted to give Judith something. I hopped off my bike and dove into my hamper to retrieve the green hospital jammies she'd worn to my transplant.

"Here!" I cried joyously. "These'll look great with a little Gap T-shirt."

The sad thing is – I meant it.

As Judith left, my friend David arrived from San Francisco. Having been diagnosed with lymphoma in 1974, David knew exactly what I needed, from morphine to massage. For the first couple of days, when he wasn't attending to my physical needs, we watched one perfect movie after another – *Harold and Maude, The Big Chill, Hannah and Her*

Sisters, A Thousand Clowns – laughing in the sad parts, crying in the happy. It was a happy time, when nothing else mattered – we were alive.

By day three, however, the honeymoon was over. My euphoria was gone – replaced by fever, nausea and the kind of sore throat where you just keep swallowing because you're so afraid of the pain you're about to endure you want to hurry up and see if you'll survive.

When I wasn't busy swallowing, I was taking my temperature, terrified that my fever would shoot up even higher, at which point they would give me more antibiotics in a kind of hit-or-miss attempt to control whatever infection might be causing it. Since by now my white blood count was down to zero, the notion of hit-or-miss was not very reassuring. I also dreaded the side effects of the antibiotics they might give me, such as Amphotericin, nicknamed "Amphoterrible" and "Shake and Bake" for its side effects of chills and *more* fever.

And then there were rules for *avoiding* infection. These had to be followed *at all costs.* I could do nothing that might break my skin, even unnoticeably. Now that I had no white blood cells to fight infection and very few platelets to help me clot, simple acts that I'd always taken for granted – brushing my teeth, opening my mail, filing my nails, blowing my nose – could kill me.

So I brushed my teeth with little "Toothettes" – soft, pink, spongy things that look like what you'd use to wash dollhouse dishes. Somebody else opened my mail. My nails, well, they just grew off the map. And my nose, my nose – God, my nose drove me crazy. Not being able to blow it was like having an itch that *no one* could scratch.

Early one morning, before David arrived, my nose just

sort of started running. Which reminded me of my favorite Martin Mull line, "Noses run in my family," which made me kind of laugh/snort, which made my nose run some more, which made me want to blow it so badly I could (you should pardon the expression) taste it. I decided to take a piece of Kleenex and just pat it; after all, that wouldn't exactly be "blowing," per se. But once that Kleenex got in the vicinity, oh, God, please forgive me, I gave the eensy weensy teensiest honk and, before I knew it, my nose was blown.

When David arrived, I blurted with a mixture of glee and relief: "I blew my nose!" But then he glared at me like a father catching his three-year-old using a chain saw to slice a bagel, and I knew I was in trouble.

"You *what?*" he screeched, Police of Infection, Deputy of Blood.

I was so ashamed of breaking the rule that out of my mouth fell – with the innocence and intensity of a child who once told me that her "pencil made a mistake and broke" – what I, under pressure, believed to be TRUTH. "I don't know what happened, David; my nose, it just blew itself."

Hearing me blame my nose for attempted murder, we both broke into prolonged fits of laughter – causing my nose to blow itself again.

And *this* moment, I'm sorry to report, was the highlight of my transplant.

❧

After David came Marilyn, his wife, my friend of thirty years and the original "Pointless Sister" who'd been flown in for my birthday party and who'd been living with breast cancer since 1982. We talked and talked for hours on end.

About the past – "Crud Savage" and "Harvey Fingers." About the present – cancer, baldness, chemo, men, music, art, theatre, food. But never, not once, did we mention the future.

After Marilyn came Marcia, my friend since 1968 when we met on a tour bus in Jerusalem, the only two laughing (out of guilt-peppered pity) at the tour guide's horrible jokes. Sadly, Marcia had this hospital thing down to an all-too-perfect science, her mother having recently died of ovarian cancer.

Joni returned as Marcia left. Mindy returned as Joni left. Steffie returned as Mindy left. Dale returned as Steffie left. Bobbi came. Cheryl came. The chain of visitors didn't quit. People were being wait-listed. And time became something I measured in blood counts, fevers, visits, and mail.

As weeks went on, I began to wonder why everyone who visited said, "You're doing great," no matter what. Finally I discovered that Joni, Harriet, and my sister Carol had lovingly, obsessively authored a manual of instructions for all who would come: ". . . she *must* do her mouth care four times a day . . . don't let her trick you into giving her food . . . tell her you love her, she's doing great . . . and, by all means, never give her blue gowns. Only the green ones with the little dots . . ."

Time telescoped. Days blurred. I'd wake up with *Lucy*, eat ice chips with *The Brady Bunch* and ride my bike with *Trapper John*. Then I'd drag myself to the door, press my nose to the wired-glass window, and wait in my cage for a nurse to arrive with the results from tests on blood snatched from my body during "Mean-Old-Mr.-Middle-of-the-Night." Like a four-year-old at the end of the day, waiting for Daddy to round the corner.

My primary nurse, Ann – the best on the planet – would bring me my zero white-blood-cell counts each day with love and reassurance: "This takes time. This is normal." Nonetheless, the rest of my time was spent wondering if the God of White Blood Cells would dare pass me by.

Occasionally, Ann would bring me a note from Dryden – my blood brother from pheresis – who was alive and well and pulling out his remaining three hairs in the room next to mine. With all the visitors I was allowed to have, I couldn't visit Dryden and he couldn't visit me. So we wrote back and forth, joking about marrying each other when the war was behind us, registering for dishes in the hospital gift shop and, of course, competing fiercely for the most and best white blood cells ever.

Dryden won. When he was discharged, a week earlier than I, he gave me a gift – a coffee mug that says, "I can't do a thing with my hair. Hell, I can't even find it." If you're reading this, Dryden, wherever you are, thanks, I love you and I hope you're thriving.

It was Ann who woke me one sunny morning, almost six weeks after I'd been admitted, and handed me a piece of paper. "I'm not on duty yet," she said. "But I had to be here to see your face."

The paper indicated that, overnight, my number of "mature" white blood cells (the kind that are ready to fight infection) had increased 700 percent! All things being equal, I was ready to go home. It was then that I told Ann I'd changed my name to Fanny.

Ann came to spend the morning with me the day I was discharged, even though it was her day off – the only one she would have for weeks. She brought me a gift "for going out into the world." It was perfect – a pen and pencil set engraved with my new name.

PART THREE

OUT OF THE BEDPAN INTO THE FIRE

Ten

❦

Sitting on the airplane, hot and suffocating under my face mask, flinching when anyone sneezed, I went over the rules – *No fresh fruits; No fresh vegetables; No fresh flowers; Everything well cooked; No pets; No large crowds; No young children; Only safe sex* – chanting them, silently, to the whir of the engines, unable to find the appropriate rhythm for *No walking near construction sites.* While my white blood count had climbed high enough to spring me from isolation, it needed to be higher still before I could live like a true civilian. So it was scary coming back to the real world. Everyone on the plane was an enemy because everyone on the plane had germs.

With very little twisting of my arm, Joni had persuaded me to come to Chicago to recuperate from the transplant. Since I'd lived there in the '70s, before moving to L.A., I still had plenty of Chicago friends; it would feel like home. Already I had located a furnished apartment for August and September in the area of Chicago that compares itself to New York's Soho. There was an indoor pool in my building, so I could swim every day and build myself up.

While I ate my airplane meal — fretting over whether the fruit was "canned enough" — my restriction chant went on automatic; it was snagged in my mind like an unwanted jingle: *No fresh fruits; No fresh vegetables; No fresh flowers; Everything well cooked; No pets; No large crowds; No young children; Only safe sex . . .*

A friend of Joni's, a limousine driver named Allan, would be meeting me at the airport. I would recognize him by the sign he'd be holding. He would recognize me by the *breath* I'd be holding — and if that didn't work, by my surgical mask and my floppy print hat, with no hair hanging out.

When the plane finally arrived, they let me off first to avoid the crowd of passengers. I walked through the jetway alone, feeling much like an astronaut landing on earth, trembling and chanting — *No fresh fruits; No fresh vegetables; No fresh flowers; Everything well cooked; No pets; No large crowds; No young children; Only safe sex* — still looking for the right rhythm for construction sites.

Then, on entering the airport proper — I screamed.

The terminal was gutted and under construction. It was thronged with people. And Allan was waiting with a bouquet of flowers and a basket of fruit . . .

Simple things — like taking a walk, like no more catheters, like semi-fresh air, like shopping for hats — any of these could make me cry for the first couple of weeks I was back in the world.

One particular Friday night, I was reaping the benefits of all these things, having taken a walk in the semi-fresh air with no more catheters to buy a new hat. A magnificent hat, like the one Meg Ryan wore in *When Harry Met Sally*: floppy and tilted, with a bow and rosette. And now I was home taking a bath, with my wig on, anchored beneath this gorgeous new hat. There the wig, which had always looked like a hair helmet, looked for the first time like *real* hair – beautiful hair – Kathleen Turner-sexy hair. With one side hanging half over my eye, I felt pretty for the first time in way too many months.

Afraid that if I took the wig and hat off I'd never be able to arrange them quite as perfectly, I'd decided to sweat it out in the tub with both in place. Now, as I pictured myself – buck-naked, except for my hat, splashing about in my gardenia bath – I laughed, cried, thought of Randy Newman's song "You Can Leave Your Hat On," and dialed up my fantasies to a sexy soirée.

Never good at zipless, nameless, faceless sex, I wracked my brain to picture Jack, that cutie I'd gone out with seven months prior, on the night before my hair fell out. Squinting my eyes into soft focus, I placed him in the tub: hairy chest, bulging pecks, no hat, facing me. Then, locking onto his subterranean blue eyes, I tried to get him to say his lines – stuff like "God, you're gorgeous!" and "Oooh, baby, you make me hot." But all I could get was a hyena laugh and "Why's all that sweat pouring from your wig?"

Evicting Jack from his place in the tub – and his place in my heart – I lifted my salty self from the water, thinking, "Screw fantasy; I'll swish up my lashless little peepers and take myself out for a *realistic* meal."

Joni had bought me false eyelashes – the individual one-lash-at-a-time kind, as opposed to the whole spider in one full clump – in case I ever felt inclined. As I had never used same, the next two hours were more frustrating than trying to thread a needle in the dark during an earthquake. I had lashes on my fingers, lashes on my nose – at least four false tries to every one that landed on my actual lids. Eventually, though, I must admit, my eyes looked alive for the first time in months.

After adding some eyeliner, blush and cinnamon lipstick, I was finally able to move on to wardrobe – my new paisley corduroy jodhpurs, my new olive-green cotton sweater, my new/old/but never-before-worn thirties tweed jacket (from a store called Flashy Trash) and my latest present from Joni – fabulous Ralph Lauren brown lace-up boots. The jodhpur look made me feel sexy. Tonight, perhaps, I would find a man. If I didn't find a man, a horse would do.

But walking and whistling through the Not-So-Windy City, blissing out on the mid-August air, I became more involved with what I could find to eat that wouldn't kill me than how I would find Mr. Right (or Mr. Ed). What was I whistling? Yes, of course, that snappy little number – *No fresh vegetables . . . Everything well cooked . . . No large crowds . . . Only safe sex . . . .* And, before I knew it, my whistling had carried me to my favorite Indian restaurant, where everything would be *way* overcooked and where it was so uncrowded as to be empty, except for one other diner. And this was a man who, from out of the corner of my eye, appeared to be a perfect contender for my next Mr. Wrong – thinning long hair and compensatory beard, shiny fair face, sparkling blue eyes and a matching blue work shirt unbuttoned to the heart, revealing a heavenly, hairy chest.

He was seated alone at a little banquette, back against the wall, facing east. I was seated alone at a little banquette, back against the wall, facing west. About twelve feet of dining area, two tables deep, was all that lay between us. He was drinking a martini, so I ordered some wine. His appetizers looked great – Indian bread, some yogurt spread, some lentils, some chutney. So I ordered same, except for the spread, which contained killer cukes, lethal onions and suicide dill. Then I pulled out a book and, holding it at table's length, started to read, squinting attractively so as not to see double, having realized that, in order to put on my wire-rimmed glasses, I'd need to remove my hat and wig.

After reading the same sentence twenty times, I looked over at Mr. Maybe to see if perhaps he was looking at me. The answer was – maybe. Embarrassed that he might've seen me looking to see if he was looking at me, I hastily returned to my book and began to devour my appetizers and wine.

Three chapters to the wind by the time my Tandoori chicken arrived, our main course got a little juicier. Since distance was the strong suit of my failing vision, I could see across the room to his mixed-grill plate and his Burgundy wine. The place was quickly filling up, and it was getting tricky to stay in his line of sight, but I did my best, eating with manners that had grown pretty rusty during hospital life and praying he wasn't looking when I used my knife as a mirror, about every third bite, to see if my mixed vegetables had landed in my teeth, if my lipstick had made it to my chin, if my wig had chosen to slip, if my lashes were still on my lids. Finally, somewhere between my Tandoori breast and my Tandoori thigh, our eyes locked – but only for a second – during which time I got up the guts to flash my victim a blushingly vulnerable "I'm available" smile. Feeling, at last, that my groundwork was done, that contact had been made, I could now relax with the rest of my food and reflect over what, if anything, had just happened.

Had I actually just flirted? Did I even remember how? When was the last time I'd done such a thing? At least two years ago; probably longer. What did I look like to this total stranger? It was one thing to be feeling attractive in a relative way, having rigged up a wig and lashed up my eyes after so many months of baldness, floppy hats, giant earrings, and well-meaning loved ones saying, "You look great." But this guy had no prior notion of me to help enhance what I'd accomplished. And even if he found what he *saw* attractive, how would he like me – disassembled?

My coffee came. I sipped it slowly, trying to stall while he finished his meal. But just as I reached the bottom of my cup, the waiter brought him another course – some vegetable mush. What a pig. So I ordered dessert – "Gulab Jamam," little round balls of cake soaked in honey that taste like the lining of your grandmother's purse.

When I finished, *he* was on *his* coffee. I didn't want more coffee, but I needed something to do, so I played Tea Party, pouring pretend coffee from my empty silver pot into my empty cup, pretend-sipping as I read my book. I checked on him again after several minutes, when I figured he'd probably be getting his check. But no; now Mr. Forget-It was sipping a liqueur. "That's it," I thought, paying my check, adjusting my wig and hefting myself from too long at the table. "The rest is up to the powers that be."

On the way out, however, passing his table, I couldn't

help but say, "Nice eating with you."

One beat later, a voice from behind caught up with me. "Wait," he called. "I'm coming with you."

He, it turned out, had kept *his* food coming in an attempt to smoothly exit with *me*.

Out on the street he said, "Where are we going?"

"To Paris," I answered, and led him through the balmy streets to my favorite little outdoor café.

❧

Backlit by a street lamp, up close and personal, Dennis was even more attractive now that we'd moved from India to France. The café was filled with dark, thin, exotic people, chain-smoking and speaking French.

"I see why you said 'Paris,'" Dennis observed. "All that's missing is the stench of the *pissoir*."

"I can take you to the bus station if you really miss it."

"Or *I* can take *you* to France."

We got lost in the dream. After all, we both had our passports and American Express cards. What else did we need? We'd get up from the table, head to the airport, hold each other all the way to France, then let fate and the magic of the Paris Métro carry us the rest of the way. I didn't tell Dennis what was keeping me from going – a low white blood count and the need to be close to a doctor I trusted. I let *his* excuse cover us both – in town from New York to deliver a paper; they were counting on him; he couldn't jump ship.

As the evening unfolded it became more apparent that this was a man who could *never* jump ship. A divorced, joint-custody father of two, working seventeen-hour days as an intensive-care doctor, he clearly had time for little else. He *did* have a second home in Woodstock, where he hinted we might go, sometime, if I'd like. *If I'd like!*

My mind was whirring. Here was Mr. Absolutely Perfect. An intensive-care doctor – he could keep me alive. A father of two – I could have children without having children. A home in Woodstock – a place I could write. And he'd be so tired, and so-o-o-o absent, he'd fill my deep neurotic need – to always be needing *more*.

We talked for hours, mostly about him, because I wasn't ready to reveal my tale. We were hitting it off; we were both clearly smitten; I was scared the whole thing would go up in smoke if he knew I'd just had a transplant.

When we left the café, we walked along the lake, holding hands and reminiscing about how we had met – so long ago.

"Wouldn't this be a great story to tell our grandchildren?" Dennis said, squeezing my hand. What *exactly* did he mean by that? I didn't dare ask; I was too terrified. Instead I asked him, "When did you know you wanted to know me?"

"The minute you walked through the restaurant door."

"How could you tell?"

"The hat."

"The hat?"

"Anyone with the style and chutzpah to wear that hat, I knew had to have some brains to match." (Shit, here we go; another guy after me for my brains.)

"Can I see you tomorrow night?" Dennis asked.

"No, shoot, I'm busy tomorrow night." The thought of missing a moment with this man felt like archery to my heart.

"How about Saturday, during the day?"

"I can't," I responded, pouting by now. "But Saturday *night* I'm free."

"Great," he said, then fired another arrow. "I'll be leaving Chicago Sunday at noon."

Was it too soon to say, "I'll go home with you – I don't live in Chicago, I don't live in L.A., I'm a *tabula rasa*, I can move to New York – as long as you monitor my blood count, that is, as long as you keep me alive"?

In the cab, on the way home, we had our first kiss. A sweet, gentle, tentative kiss that opened the steel gates of my heart to a yearning, a longing that cut so deep I actually almost threw up.

We got out of the cab, then stayed together for a while in front of my building, hugging goodnight. Dennis wanted to come up; I wanted to slow *down*. I was much too anxious, with fast-forward fantasies that were driving me wild plus a paralyzing fear that he'd disappear as soon as he knew the truth.

As we kissed one more time, Dennis caressed what he thought was my hair, making me even *more* anxious, then looked in my eyes and lovingly said, "Yes, anyone with a hat like that . . ."

"Look!" I stopped him. "I've got something to tell you." If he was going to run, I wanted him to do it now.

"I wasn't going to tell you," I said. "Not yet; I was afraid if I did, you wouldn't see me again."

"What on earth could you possibly tell me that would make me not want to see you again?"

"Try this on for size. The reason I'm wearing the hat is it's holding on my wig. The reason I'm wearing the wig is I had a transplant for breast cancer. I'm two weeks out of transplant. I'm recuperating in Chicago. My home is L.A. I might not go back there. I might stay *here*. I might not make it. I'm not a great bet."

Without skipping a beat, Dennis responded, "How could you possibly think that would matter?"

"Please," I said, as relief flooded me (with an undertow of doubt). "You're a doctor!"

"You've just had one of the most advanced treatments. State of the art. You're going to be fine."

"Right," I answered, still not convinced.

He kissed me again, and held me for the longest time. But not long enough. Then he hailed a cab and, as he left, hollered, "See you Saturday. I still love your hat."

I wished, in that moment, I had the nerve to toss it in the air like Mary Tyler Moore.

The reason I couldn't see Dennis Friday night or Saturday afternoon was that I'd previously signed up to attend a seminar on healing with a man named Brugh Joy. I'd heard about Brugh for several years from friends claiming they knew people who'd gone to him on their last legs and were still around to tell the story. In the past, my skepticism had outweighed my curiosity; now the reverse was true.

Brugh Joy had been a medical doctor until 1974, when his own life-threatening illness moved him to give up his practice and explore other areas of healing – areas involving body energies, meditation, and higher levels of consciousness. In short, all the stuff that, until I met him, I'd always referred to as "Hoogie Moogie." But now – what did I have to lose?

On Friday, for good luck, I wore the jodhpur outfit in which I'd met Dennis, complete with wig and hat. That evening, Brugh introduced us to some of his ideas, then mapped out how we'd be working the next day. There were two hundred people. The atmosphere was warm. And my outfit was useless.

On Saturday morning Brugh worked with three volunteers, one at a time, in front of the rest of us, using their dreams to slice through their psyches. As he gently unfolded their patterns and conflicts, celebrating their many "selves" – opening the door to transformation and healing – I was mesmerized.

In the afternoon Brugh would be working with two more volunteers, using disease as he'd earlier used dreams. If you wanted to be one of them, you had to put your name in a bucket along with those of all the others there who were literally dying for a moment with Brugh. Brugh would choose the two names. My pen quickened. I wanted a moment with him as much as I'd wanted my transplant – like ice cream on top of the pie.

I noticed, when I put my name down, that I automatically wrote "Jill." Even my "Hello-My-Name-Is" tag said "Jill." Fanny obviously hadn't jelled. I decided to put both names in the bucket; that way I'd have twice the chance of being picked. More importantly – if Brugh picked "Fanny," I'd know it was time to get serious about her. (In my deepest, darkest secret heart, I'd also decided that, if he picked me, I'd live.)

I was sorry I hadn't worn my good-luck outfit when Brugh pulled "Chuck" from the bucket. The two of them did amazing work up there on the stage. It was painful. It was moving. We needed a break.

After the break, I was so busy chatting with someone I'd just met that I didn't hear Brugh announce: "Fanny Gaynes, prepare yourself."

Someone nudged me. "Isn't that you?"

"Huh?"

"Fanny Gaynes?" Brugh summoned once more.

Oh, my God! My prayers had been answered. Pie *à la mode*. I flew to the stage in my *new* "good luck" outfit – jeans, no wig, and my floppy print hat.

❧

"Obviously, her unconscious makes a statement." Those were his first words about me. "She may think she's in charge of it, but it's a very powerful force."

He proceeded to show me just *how* powerful, through a terrifying, yet gentle and ultimately exquisite unfolding of some of my hidden selves.

It didn't take long for Brugh to get to one of the most painful of these selves. This was the part of me who's always been angry at being a girl, who's never felt nurtured, who's never felt loved, who's so afraid of her deep, deep longings – so doubtful of her ability to love and be loved – that she runs from men who mirror her neediness and seeks out men who mirror her fears, avoiding commitment at all costs. Yes, the part of me who would rather *die* than give up her freedom, who finally confessed: "If I die I won't ever have to grow up."

The picture was bleak. I was in tears; the audience was in shock.

But we went on, and I talked about my stem-cell transplant. And Brugh turned to the audience and said, "So now we're beginning to see and *feel* the immense power of another part of her, another part of her that seeks life, that seeks to go through a horrendous – I mean, talk about *horrendous* – initiation." Describing "the immense suffering that goes on when one is that vulnerable," he said to me:

"Tell us what that feels like to you right now."

"What I'm responding to," I said softly, through tears, " . . . is how much I *do* want to live. I really like it here. I think it's a fun place."

"Now this is *another* part of her," Brugh said, laughing, " . . . the part that's speaking that it *is* fun. There are other parts of her in there also. But what I'm after . . . is, obviously, the one that really has street survival instincts." He saw "street savvy" in me, he said, survival forces that were "very powerful."

There was a part of me that wanted life just because it was afraid of death, he said. But beyond that was "another quality . . . There's a richer woman underneath all of this that really has never had a chance to live, and it seeks something – to express more fully that it understands the mystery of near-death and it's time for its, sort of like, place in the sun . . .

"Although all of these patterns are active within you – and they're immortal patternings – the one that I'm interested in is: Where is the one that is giving you life *now?*"

To the gathering Brugh said: "We must not be afraid to see the forces that are leading to her life and the forces that are leading to her death – because they're still in there." If I could acknowledge and welcome these many aspects of my self, he said, I would find that the vulnerable, fearful parts could be cared for by the stronger ones. He went on: "If you were to state what fulfills you at this point in your life, giving you a sense of connectedness to whatever the life spirit is, what would you say is meaningful to you – at *this* point?"

"My friendships," I answered. "That's the big meat and potatoes for me. And writing."

"Meat and potatoes," Brugh repeated. Then, to the audience, "I have to listen to this now, because meat and potatoes is usually masculine . . ."

"That's the big cookie?" I asked.

Brugh laughed. "No – 'Meat and Potatoes,' *he's* in there; he's probably got a big burly chest. And *he* values friendship too. But you know, the psyche can change from part to part very fast. So there's 'Meat and Potatoes' in there, but I'm also fascinated by the fact that you've chosen a very interesting name. Fanny." He repeated it slowly. "Fa-a-n-ny. Fanny has a lot of play and force in it. It also has a lot of psychosexuality in it.

"The 'Fanny' is very different than – what *is* his name? . . . 'Meat and Potatoes' – the *him* in you. Do you have a name for him?"

Actually, I did, I told him – in fact, two names. They were what my father called me just when I was "blossoming" in adolescence: Butch or Sam.

"Butch or Sam! Do you hear that?" Brugh cried. "Do you hear the word Butch in 'butcher?' Do you hear that material there?" As he continued to speak, I began to understand –and to *feel* – some of the ways in which this masculine aspect of me had come to dominate other aspects, even squashing them into invisibility. Fanny, bless her heart – *my* heart – was a part who wouldn't be squashed.

But Brugh now was cautioning us against blaming those parts of ourselves that may have hindered us, and against blaming other people for how we had grown. "The richness comes in understanding a much larger context of life and being, other than the one that talks about '*My parents did this to me,*'" he said, "because they *didn't.*" He went on to describe his belief that "the material was struck at conception . . . and what elicits responses from parents and other people is tied into fundamental patterns that we carry, that we cannot divorce ourselves from." For me, he said, "the fundamental issue of her confusion around male and female was part of the wondrous, mysterious hand that she's been dealt to live *through.* For that is one of the great patternings in life . . . that leads to immense resource – if we can ever mature *through* it."

Brugh looked at me. "Do you know what I'm talking about?"

"Yes." I was crying. "This is a really wonderful moment. Thank you."

"Yes, it is," he answered. "It really is. Because it's bringing you to something about Butch and Sam inside . . . and Fanny, who's finally getting out a little bit.

"And I can tell you," he added, as he looked to the audience, "Fanny isn't a little girl. Fanny knows how to wear a boa."

There are no adequate earthly words to describe how I felt as I returned to the planet after being cracked open by Brugh. Born? Raw? Vulnerable? Trusting? Loving? Mad? Joyful? Big? Teeny? Dead? Alive? Totally awake? All of the above.

I only had an hour between returning from Brugh at 5:00 and seeing Dennis at 6:00. What I needed was a decompression chamber. What I settled for was a bath.

In the tub, very carefully shaving my legs, I laughed remembering a night ten years back when I felt so ambivalent about whether to have sex with my boyfriend that I only shaved one leg. This was definitely a two-leg night.

When Dennis arrived, exactly on time, I felt radiant in another version of the jodhpur look – this time, taupe, wide-wale corduroy jodhpurs, a beautiful, soft, off-white sweater, gargantuan earrings I'd bought at the conference (kind of gold-meshy-lacy-dangly, surrounding a cameo, *très femme*) and, of course, my wig and famous hat. Our greeting was sweet and nervous.

Out on the street, walking to dinner, holding hands, we both relaxed and Dennis told me about his day. His paper was well received; he'd finished at noon, spent some time at the lake, had a Chicago pizza, then headed back to his hotel for a sauna and massage. There was no way I could rattle off *my* day like that, so I told him the bottom line – my name was now Fanny, though he'd met me as Jill.

At dinner, in a romantic Japanese restaurant, Dennis admitted he'd been thinking about me ever since we met.

"It's so confusing and wonderful," he said, "to be sitting here in a new city with a total stranger who I feel like I've known all my life."

I wanted to have at his hairy chest.

"It made me so sad," he went on, "to see your anguish over the thought of my reaction to your cancer."

Now I wanted him – just to hold me. Tight. Till the day I died.

"You have to go on with your life," he continued, as tears began to run down my face. "People aren't going to run from you. You have to believe that. You have to know."

My heart exploded. I jumped up, ran to the bathroom, locked myself in and slid to the floor. There, sobbing, trembling, rocking, gasping, I tried to take myself in hand.

It's horrible, I thought, *wanting something so much.* Especially a man. Wanting a transplant, wanting to live – that was O.K.. But wanting a *man* – as much, it seemed in that moment, as I'd wanted to live – that was *not* O.K. with me. Still I couldn't stop shaking. I couldn't stop rocking. I felt like a junkie; I wanted my fix – even though I knew that nothing could *fix* me. Especially Dennis.

A woman knocking on the bathroom door finally brought me back to earth. With a quick repair job to my falsely lidded eyes, and my falsely lidded head, I returned to Dennis and my glass of plum wine.

"Are you all right?" he asked.

"Who me?" I laughed – a too-hard laugh, the kind you hear on the psycho ward. "I'm sorry, Dennis. I'm off the map."

I wanted him to know me – right away. All of me. *Now.* The whole truth. *Fast.* I thought of my most adored Uncle Ernie, an exquisite man with a passion for life, who'd been battling cancer for thirty-seven years. Whenever the family didn't move fast enough for him, on some excursion or another, he'd yell, "C'mon, everyone. Hurry! Can't you see? I'm in a desperate race against time."

"Speaking of being off the map," Dennis was saying, "what's to become of us anyway?"

"Huh?"

"I mean, you're in Chicago. I'm in New York. And with the hours that I work and my life with my kids, I can't visit *you* and, if you come to visit me, we'll be grabbing an hour here and there and maybe, if we really push it, every fifth week, an entire day."

"Why are we talking about this *now*?" I asked.

"Because that's what I've been thinking about ever since we met."

I melted. And he went on: "I've only had one experience with a long-distance relationship. And it was a total disaster."

Funny, I thought. My best relationships were always long distance; being apart was what kept us together. "So what are you saying?" I asked.

"I don't know. I'm just voicing my fears and doubts, I suppose. I'm not sure it's anything we can resolve in an evening."

(C'mon. Hurry! Can't you see? I'm in a desperate race against time.)

After dinner we went for a walk; a quiet, tender, arms-around-each-other walk. Eventually, wending our way toward my apartment, we stopped at a convenience store and bought all the makings for an orgy – Ben & Jerry's ice cream, patchouli incense, a single rose, and a lifetime supply of condoms (three).

Back at my place, we cracked open the ice cream and, high on our scoops of Chunky Monkey, waddled our way to my king-size bed. How I managed what followed amazes me to this day. Off came my lovely off-white sweater and matching off-white shoulder pads. Off came my bra and my "life-like" prosthesis. Off came my jodhpurs and bikini undies – leaving me once again buck-naked except for my earrings, my hat and my wig.

Then – "Fuck it," I said, in a moment of passion, and tossed my hat and wig on the lamp, actually believing that leaving my earrings would call attention away from my head.

What followed is a blur in memory. Somehow we made love, but it felt like razor blades (no one had warned me that chemo can turn you into sandpaper "down there").

Dennis, for all practical purposes, was long gone before we were done. We didn't talk about it; just fell asleep – that sleep where the man snores all night and the woman dozes in and out of intrapsychic pain.

In the morning, I asked what he was feeling. "Numb," he said. Not a good sign.

Dennis left me with a perfunctory kiss, heading back to his hotel to pack. He'd return in an hour for a perfunctory brunch. As I closed the door behind him, the feeling in my stomach reminded me of a feeling I'd ignored that first night, when Dennis had said of my cancer, "How could you possibly think that would matter?" Like a shark yanking at my lower intestine, trying to tell me what I didn't want to hear – "The doctor doth protest too much."

Reassembling myself in hat, wig and equestrian look, I tried to talk myself out of my pain. *He's only a man. You don't even know him. What's the big deal? You're alive; that's what counts.* But nothing I said could fill the hole. I can hardly remember a lonelier hour.

At brunch, Dennis told me what I already knew. He just couldn't do it; he couldn't take the chance. *What* chance? I thought. That I'd die before the relationship did? That I'd out*live* the relationship? Perhaps a little of both.

He was all of my love affairs – all my goodbyes.

And I was his kiss of death.

Eleven

❦

The next day, still reeling from the beauty of Brugh and the disaster of Dennis, I went shopping with my old friend Alex. Tall, elegant and superbly intelligent, Alex always reminded me of Alan Alda without the quirkiness. He and I had been lovers in 1972. I had just returned from Vietnam, deeply wounded by the war between me and my boyfriend, a foreign correspondent whom I'd gone over to marry and didn't. Alex was working on his Ph.D. in French literature and was in the beginning stages of splitting from both his wife and his life as an Orthodox Jew. He taught me religion; I taught him McDonald's.

Alex and I spent a month or two believing that our love could transcend our neuroses. Never before and never since have I been in a relationship that involved so much rage. We were always screaming; we were never heard. We had no idea what our anger was about. When it became clear that Alex wasn't ready to leave his wife, I left the relationship, disguising as the "sane" one who *would* have committed – if only.

After enough time had passed, we ran into each other and, without the heat and pressure of romance, were able to become friends.

Alex lived in Chicago, and it was wonderful to be near him again. We'd been going to dinners and movies, taking walks, talking a lot on the telephone and generally having fun. Now we were on an excursion to Bloomingdale's. I, of course, needed hats and jodhpurs; he needed some clothes and a suitcase for a trip he was planning. A salesperson, showing us some luggage, mentioned that "this one comes with a five-year guarantee."

Out of my mouth tumbled, "I wish *I* came with a five-year guarantee."

Alex gave me a look, told the woman he'd think about the luggage, then whisked me off to a place in Bloomies where we could have a cup of coffee.

"I hate when you talk like that," he said to me over double espresso and chocolate biscotti.

"Like what?" I'd already forgotten what I'd been saying, now that the chocolate had found its way home.

"Like you wish *you* came with a five-year guarantee."

"Well, I *do*," I said and my eyes began to brim.

"Look, kiddo, you're going to be fine. I know this sounds crazy, but I *know* you'll be fine; it's *not* your time; you're *not dying*. Not now and not for a long time. In fact, you'll probably outlive me."

There aren't many people who can get away with talking to me that way. Dennis had, but only because I wanted so much for things to work out between us. If I'd trusted what my stomach told me that first night, I'd have known he was speaking from his own denial and fear of death. Which is fine; we all have it. But the truth is: When your life is really threatened —when you actually might be dying — *there is nothing worse* than to have someone telling you you're not. It's painful; it's lonely; it's not being *seen.* Tell me you *don't know* what's going to happen to me; tell me it doesn't *feel* like I'm dying; tell me any variation on the theme, but don't flat out tell me I'm *not.*

Unless, that is, you've been given permission.

Joni had been given permission. She'd earned it through a long, trusting, knowing friendship laced with a tremendous amount of humor and a psychic connection so deep that there were actually times she'd be vomiting in Chicago while I was getting chemo in L.A. It was Joni who — hearing me pop out of bed in the middle of the first night after my diagnosis — knew to yell from the other room, "What are we doing, darling? Estate planning?" Bingo.

And, when I was struggling through the transplant, it was Joni who could say — firmly, teeth-clenchedly, with total conviction — "*YOU ARE GOING TO MAKE IT.*"

"I am?" I would ask her, sheepishly.

"*YES, YOU ARE!*"

"Really?"

"*YES-S-S-S-S.*"

"You're not just saying that because I've got cancer?"

"*STOP IT! YOU'RE GOING TO BE FINE.*"

"Yes?"

"*YES!*"

And I actually believed her. But that was because I'd *chosen* Joni, through unspoken contract, to be my coach. *I* believed Joni because *Joni* believed Joni. Where *my* strength left off, *hers* took over; then she'd feed it back to me. That's what coaches do. And that's what helped to pull me through.

So here I was with Alex telling me the same thing, and I guess because I'd always seen him as mystical, magical, knowing and wise – I believed him. At least I believed that *he* truly believed I was going to live. That he wasn't just pacifying me. That I wasn't just hearing a pretty disguise for his own fear, his own denial. In other words, Alex had been "given permission."

"Thanks, Alex, for telling me that."

He gave me a sweet little crooked smile, then asked, "So what have you been up to lately?"

"Well, this past weekend, I'd venture to say, I had the most amazing experience of my entire life."

"Oh, yeah?" His moustache twitched.

"God, I don't know where to start. Have you ever heard of Brugh Joy?"

"No, I don't think so."

"Well, Brugh Joy is a spiritual healer, a layer-on of hands, a transformational therapist . . . and in that particular circle, he's one of the best."

"According to whom? *Consumer Reports*?"

I let the barb pass, but it cut like a knife.

"So what happened?" Alex asked.

I told him about the dreamwork Brugh did. Then I told him about putting both my names, Jill and Fanny, into the bucket and how Brugh picked Fanny out of *all* those people.

Alex's comment was: "Uh-huh."

I got quiet.

"So then what happened?" he asked, in an uninterested tone.

"You know what?" I said, as kindly as I could. "I think it'd be better if I tell you about this another time."

"Are you angry with me?" he asked.

Well, I hadn't thought so, but now that he mentioned it . . ."Yes, Alex, I guess I *am* angry with you."

"Well, how do you know I'm not angry with *you* too?"

"Jesus, Alex, if you're angry with *me*, just tell me; don't ask me if *I'm* angry with you and then throw it back in my face."

"So why are you angry, anyway?" he pursued.

"Because sometimes you're so self-absorbed. Here I'm spilling a story to you that's changed my life and all I get is a bad joke and a couple of 'uh-huhs' and suddenly I just don't feel like going on."

"Self-absorbed!" Alex screamed. "*Self-absorbed! You're* calling *me* self-absorbed? You're the most self-absorbed person I've ever known. I'm sick of walking on eggshells with you! I have needs too."

"What would you like from me?" I asked him.

"If I have to tell you, then what's the point?" (Always my favorite – the mind-reader fight.) "Self-absorbed!" he exclaimed a few more times, then capped his complaint:

"I'm sorry *I'm* not dying of cancer, but *I* have problems too."

Now, I understood that I'd become so obsessed with my disease, there were times I could see nothing else. I understood that Alex "had problems too" – serious problems: that he suffered from depression, and that facing depression is like facing death.

Unfortunately, though, Alex's anger had unlocked his truth – he saw me as dying. And I could not be around someone who saw me as dying. Not for a second. Not *then.* Not *now.*

❧

Sitting at home, stunned by how quickly a seventeen-year friendship can go down the toilet, I was totally absorbed in the question of whether I was actually as self-absorbed as Alex had said. Then the mail arrived and saved my day. It brought an article that had been written by my friend Marcia for a Long Island paper called *The Women's Record.*

The headline was "Soulmates," and in it Marcia described her friendship with me, starting from our encounter on the Israeli tour bus. She wrote of our vast differences and our deep affection, and went on to tell how she had come to Nebraska to be with me at the transplant hospital.

"We spent the essence of 'quality time' together in Omaha this summer during her three-month hospital stay," Marcia had written. "There was no question that the only way I could survive her enduring what was described as 'horrific' treatment was to be there with her. Not so much because I wanted to (I'd have loved to convince myself she didn't need me, it wasn't necessary, I'd keep up by phone), but because I had to. It was much easier to handle this crisis in person than waiting and worrying. And never in my life did I get back so much for what I gave.

"Leave it to Jill, I never had to cope with what I was most afraid of. I knew I could handle the baldness, the retching, even the weakness. What I feared was her fear, her depression. I didn't count on the fact that my friend of twenty years, who I would've sworn I knew inside and out, was a closet hero.

"Her massive reserves of courage, positive thinking and the world's best sense of humor made my job easy . . . I wanted to give her what I was sure she needed (actually, what I projected I would need if I were her), a person she could 'why me?' to, someone she could rage and cry and spit out her anger to over how unfair, how despicably unfair, this life was being to her. But she was too busy making herself available to new patients who were coming in for the treatment, reassuring them how much easier it was to live through than anticipate. She was too busy opening the mail (over 200 cards arrived from her immediate world), and volunteering for tests to help with new research and helping a nurse write lyrics to a rap song for a supervisor who was retiring. It wasn't draining spending time there, it was energizing."

Thanks, pal.

The days got shorter. The nights got longer. Autumn fell into winter. And *I* fell into a funk. I can hardly remember what I did with my time. Swam, I guess; ate, I suppose; read, maybe, when I could manage to focus. I was tired from the transplant, but unwilling to admit it. I felt guilty for not wanting to smell every rose, and obsessed with the fear that my disease was still there. I was still feeling the aftereffects of the session with Brugh Joy – now being Fanny for sure, and no longer Jill except occasionally – but in this grey time even that exhilaration seemed faded.

I was being checked every two weeks by Joni's doctor at Northwestern University Medical Center. Mostly this was routine transplant follow-up stuff. But we were also watching a heaviness in my chest that could mean new disease or merely anxiety over *thoughts* of new disease. There was no way to tell yet, since lesions that are healing can look the same, upon X-ray, as persistent tumor. So the best we could hope for was no increase in *anything* from one X-ray to the next. Which turned out to be the case for my chest.

In December, however, I had some pain in my back, and X-rays revealed some "sclerotic" (hardened) areas on my spine. Since these areas had never been X-rayed before, we had no prior film with which to compare them. They could very well have been there before the transplant. But to be certain, I'd have to have a bone scan, using radioactive isotopes to "light up" any spots where tumors might be attacking the bone.

Once you're injected with isotopes, you have to wait two hours before being scanned. Joni and I filled the gap with a long, nervous breakfast during which we reviewed my life, discussed whether I would be buried in L.A. or Detroit, and debated what I should wear for my date that evening with a new man, named Norman, whom I'd met the day before.

Back at the hospital, under the scanner, I was so busy – between planning my funeral (with an MTV-style videotaped eulogy, starring *me*) and planning my wardrobe for the evening (forget the jodhpur look; it was time for a dress) – I hardly noticed when my doctor showed up.

"Look, Fanny," she said. "There are things we can do."

"What do you mean?"

"If it's in the third lumbar, we'll irradiate the third and fourth. If it's in the fourth lumbar, we'll include the fifth."

"Wait a minute," I said. "Are you telling me you *really* think this is tumor?" And I know this sounds nuts, but until that moment, even while I was planning my funeral, I was also certain – deeply certain – that everything would be fine; there was nothing "active" on my spine.

The doctor looked at me with puppy-dog eyes. Again I asked, "Do you actually think my scan is going to show tumor?"

"I think it's going to light up like a Christmas tree," she said.

And there I lay on the table as if in split-screen – a tear falling numbly from *just* my left eye as the rest of me said lightly, in the attitude of Gidget, "Gee, I hope this doesn't put a crimp in my evening."

When the scan was over, I joined Joni in the waiting room while my film was being read. Five minutes later, the doctor appeared with the most incredulous expression I'd ever seen. "My hunch was wrong, Fanny. Your bone scan is normal."

"Normal?" I cried.

"Yes," she said, with tears in her eyes.

"*Normal* normal? Like a *normal* person?"

"Yes."

"I mean like a civilian – someone who's *never* had cancer?"

"Yes," she assured me. "I'm so sorry I scared you; I've just never been so sure. I wanted to prepare you . . ."

❧

Well, a day like that was a hard act for Norman to follow. But I must give him credit. He came very close, in a sweet little romantic jazz-filled restaurant, to truly setting my soul on fire. It was hard to believe – and harder to tell him – when he didn't even notice that the menu he was reading, by candlelight, had gone up in flames, from same.

Twelve

❦

So Alex goes down in history, Norman goes up in smoke, and life, thanks to God knows what, goes on. I ring out the old year. I sing in the new. And I start to notice I have *no* desire to go back to L.A. So I find the most incredible apartment – a loft on Lake Michigan with twelve-foot, timber-beamed ceilings – and, without returning to Southern California, have movers pack me up and, as I like to say, fax me my L.A. life. Then I settle in, spend a couple of months making angels in the snow, greet the day and a half of Chicago spring and, as soon as it's summer, go out to visit friends in Northern California and scream, "Oh, my God, I meant to move *here!*"

Everything I needed was waiting for me in Marin County, about a half hour north of San Francisco. First, there was Genny Davis. She had been highly recommended, a year and a half back, as a healer/counselor whom I should definitely see. I'd always intended to, but had gotten so busy with chemo and the transplant that it hadn't yet come to pass.

Days after my arrival in the county, I had my first session with Genny. The minute she looked *through* me with her pure green eyes, the minute she touched me with those hot little hands, I said, "That does it; I'm moving here for almost sure."

That night, I dreamed that I came to a new home and on my doorstep was a housewarming gift with a card that said, "It's an Eagle Guitar; not everyone can play its notes." It was the most beautiful instrument I'd ever seen: all glass, in the shape of an eagle, with Victorian scrollwork along the edges. I held it up and the light shone through. Then I played it and notes I'd never heard before filled my mind. This was my first *pretty* dream – the first one that wasn't me in a plane that was crashing, me in a car that was exploding, or me dangling off a building on a spool of slender thread.

The next wondrous thing awaiting me was the Pine Street Clinic in San Anselmo, a place for acupuncture and herbs. As soon as I walked in I felt as if giant hands had been laid on my shoulders to guide me where I'd always belonged. New Age music, chirping birds, and babbling fountains filled the rooms. The walls of the reception area were completely lined with books, antique medicine cabinets, beautiful bottles of tonics and herbs, and all kinds of Chinese art. My appointment was with a man named McCulloch, a gentle acupuncturist/herbalist who had studied extensively in China and who interviewed me for over an hour before treating me. His acupuncture was deep; I went out almost immediately and awakened forty-five minutes later feeling peaceful, calm and extremely alive. Then he mixed up some herbs and taught me how to boil them up and take them as "tea." (This was more cooking than I'd done in years. As for the taste, two little words – "swamp" and "water" – probably sum it up best.)

Finding the Pine Street Clinic clinched the deal. In less than a week, I had been, as we like to say in the county, "Marin-ated." So I bought some wheels (Rollerblades and a mountain bike) and began my search through the towns of Marin for the perfect place to live.

There was Fairfax – charming, nestled in the hills, frozen in time – I didn't own enough tie-dye. And Mill Valley, a quaint little town beside mystical Mount Tamalpais, with curious shops and a bookstore/café where I could sip tea and work all day on this book I'd decided to write, amidst others who'd retired in their forties and taken new names – such as Chico, Rico, Duke and Sky, the first four men I actually met. Then there was Tiburon, a two-block Hollywood set of a town, right on the San Francisco Bay.

With a chain-smoking real estate agent named Sandy, I searched for apartments for an entire day and a half (in "Cancer Time," that's almost a year) and was getting discouraged by what I was finding – small, dark, boxy, uninteresting places for too much money, with too little view. I finally said to Sandy, "Listen, I'm willing to take my time; I'll live in a hotel till I find the right thing. So let me tell you what I'm looking for and don't call me until you find it." I proceeded to describe an impossible dream. "I want a studio that doesn't look like a studio; I don't know what that means, but it has to have charm – maybe part of somebody's house or something – and it has to be in Tiburon and it has to overlook something wonderful, preferably the Bay, and it has to be cheap, do you understand?"

Sandy choked on her cigarette.

When we got back to her agency, Sandy went to her office and I went next door to the shoe-repair store to salvage the day by buying some laces. In the office, Sandy was greeted by her boss, Barbara, who barked: "You didn't let Fanny go, did you? I think I've got something she'd like."

Sandy came running after me and persuaded me to come hear what Barbara had to say.

"I've never seen the place," Barbara said, "but it's a studio and it's supposed to be charming." (Sure, I thought, certain that Sandy had coached her.)

"It's behind this guy Jack's house," she continued. "He never lists it. He just tells me whenever there's going to be a vacancy and waits till I spot the perfect person."

"How do you know *I'm* the one?"

"Vibes," she answered. (Welcome to Marin.)

Barbara phoned Jack, but he wasn't home. Then, just as we'd decided to table it till the next day, the tenant who was about to move out of my alleged dream studio just *happened* to come by to say hi.

Phoebe and I hit it off right away. When I asked her to describe the apartment she said, "You need to see it to understand. If you'd like, I can take you right now."

We drove to where we couldn't go any farther or we'd be in the Bay, then turned left and started climbing through a maze-like chain of hairpin turns with breathtaking views in every direction. When we'd finally climbed as high as we could, to the top of the hill, to the end of the earth, Phoebe said: "Well, here we are."

There've been a handful of times I've been caught without words. *This* was one of them. I have traveled through

Europe and the Middle East, Southeast Asia and the U.S.A. I have seen sights *as* beautiful, but never had I seen anything *more* beautiful than what I was looking at now: an animated Monet painting on a Cinerama sky, with swirls of gently rolling fog revealing, then hiding, revealing, then hiding the San Francisco skyline, Angel Island, ferryboats, sailboats, the Golden Gate Bridge.

We walked down two flights of steps to a redwood deck that overlooked the view. Phoebe opened a door off the deck that led into the apartment. I stood in the threshold and, involuntarily, exclaimed aloud. I never really understood the expression "I thought I had died and gone to heaven" until that moment, when I found myself standing between the two worlds – and finding a place of new life. It was *exactly* the place I'd described to Sandy: a studio that didn't *look* like a studio. With four different levels and huge windows overlooking everything. With steps down into the dining and living area, steps *up* into the bedroom area, and a wonderful bathroom featuring an oversized Jacuzzi/bathtub and a giant twenty-four-paned window. There was a second, more private, deck off the living area that overlooked a fish pond, a garden, and a Japanese-style meditation house that I was welcome to use when I wanted. And then there was *all this land*; like a park, with hills and smells and wildflowers and trees and families of Bambis foraging for food.

And the rent was *less* than I'd paid in Chicago.

I looked down to see whether my jeans had become a white robe. They hadn't, so I returned to the only earthly explanation for landing in this place – I was brought here to die.

I took the place anyway, figuring everything has its price.

❦

I was actually "sitting on the dock of the Bay" at Sam's, my favorite Tiburon café, when I spotted Michael, the songwriting partner from L.A. whom "I never slept with and *could* have loved, but when *I* was married, *he* wasn't, and when *I* wasn't, *he* was." Michael, with whom the last song I'd written began: "In another life, in another time, you would've been mine."

Michael and I had spent a day together just before I went to Omaha for my transplant. We traipsed around L.A. collecting my records, closing up my business and trying desperately to pretend it was fun. As we said goodbye, with a lingering, painful, tentative hug, he devastated me by singing softly, "In another life, in another time, you would've been mine."

In our last conversation before we lost touch, when I was recuperating in Chicago, we'd been trying to locate some lyrics to a song we'd worked on. To jog our memory, Michael played an early "work tape" in which he'd gone over the melody on the piano. At one point, I heard my taped voice make a comment and was stunned at how it affected me. My body became hot and without thinking I blurted: "I'm so glad she made it, because it would absolutely break my heart to be hearing her voice if she hadn't."

And now, after all this time, there he was, as tall, lean, shiny-faced, glinty-eyed, sweet, and sexy as ever. And alone. Three tables away, he was holding a copy of *Rolling Stone* in his right hand and playing chords on his plate with his left.

My heart skipped an entire measure as I floated from my table to his. He was buried in his magazine, so I quietly sat down and waited for him to look up. When he did, all he said was: "I'm so glad you made it, because it would absolutely break my heart to be seeing you here if you hadn't."

We grabbed each other's hands, closed our eyes and said nothing for at least a minute. When his fingers began to play chords in my palms, I knew it was time to wake up.

"Where have you been? Why haven't you called? What are you doing here? God, you look great!"

"I live here now," he said.

"Me too!"

"Alone," he added.

"*Alone* alone?"

"Well, I'll always have Shawn, but Donna and I are living separately."

Shawn was his nine-year-old daughter from his first marriage; Donna, his second wife.

"Living separately? What does that mean?"

"We don't know yet. She's still in L.A. I finally couldn't stand it. I had to get out."

"Of L.A. or the marriage?"

"L.A.," he answered. (Darn, I thought.)

"Well, what about the marriage?"

"*You know. You* saw it. We want different things. The timing's all crazy. Everything's off. There's so much anger. So little trust."

"Are you hoping to work it out?"

"I don't know. First we have to get rid of the anger. If we can. Then we'll have to see what's left."

"Oh, gee, it sounds excruciating. I'm sorry." (Sorry it's not all cut-and-dried, so I can make my move.)

"Yeah, it's tough. But I love it up here. And Shawn is thriving. So's the music."

"Great," I said. "And we can finish our songs."

"Yes." Michael smiled and played a chord on my hand.

That evening we rented *When Harry Met Sally* and watched it at my place over carry-out sushi and the San Francisco Bay. After the movie, Michael held me and said, "This feels so good; I've waited so long."

"I know," I answered. "I can't believe we're *us*." Then we kissed one of those soft, sweet, slow, teasing, back and forth, endless kisses that you only see in high school or the movies.

When we finally took a break to look at each other, I said: "Well, here's the part where *I* get scared."

"Don't worry, Fanny. I'm not in a hurry."

"*I* am," I pouted. "That's the problem. And I don't want my hurry to get in our way."

"What do you mean?"

"It's my cancer, Michael. I'm fine now, but I live in its shadow . . . always running this race against time, never wanting to miss a moment. Yet I know when I rush things, they get all mucked up."

"So let's just believe we have plenty of time."

"O.K.," I agreed. "Good idea."

"But just in case, can I see you tomorrow?"

We laughed, then I answered with a kiss.

And so we began. Me and Michael. Me, Michael and Shawn. Dinners. Movies. Biking. Walks. Even work, back in the studio at great long last. And late-night talks, in which we told each other secrets we'd never even told ourselves.

Michael hadn't lied about not being in a hurry. The second time we started to become intimate, it was *he* who interrupted with "Look, I think we should talk about this."

So we talked about Donna, how their relationship was still unresolved, how he didn't want to start something with me that he might not be able to finish, how we both treasured our friendship and our working relationship and must be careful not to jeopardize either . . .

And *then* we made love. The sweetest, tenderest, tastiest, kinkiest love I've ever made.

"Are you sorry?" I asked afterward.

"No," he said. "If we hadn't done it, we would've been *talking* about *not doing it* for the next six months!"

But the next, at least, twenty times we neared lovemaking, it was Michael who'd stop us with "Look, I think we should talk about this." And I'd hear about Donna and our friendship and all that stuff again, and we'd agree not to "do it," and then we'd kiss for hours and have high school sex – everything but, and over our clothes. As if that would keep us from feeling involved.

Then, one exquisite late-autumn day, we were heading out for a bike ride on Mount Tamalpais when Michael said, "Let's stop for coffee; I've got something to tell you." So we stopped at this place with a splendid view, and that's where he told me that he and Donna were "definitely done." After which he added, "Now *I'm* scared."

"What do you mean?" I asked, jumping silently up and down in my heart.

"I realize now that Donna has been a safety net. She's kept us from getting more deeply involved. There's no more net. *That* scares me."

"What are you scared of?"

"Hurting you."

"Hurting *me*?"

"And me," he confessed. "And Shawn. What if things don't work out? Shawn adores you. I don't know how many more separations she can take."

"Don't work out with *us*?" I asked. "Or don't work out with *me*?"

"What do you mean?"

"My disease."

"I don't even think about that," Michael said.

"You don't?" I was shocked.

"No. You're so *alive*."

"Well, *I* think about it. All the time. And I'm sure I would think about it if the tables were turned."

"Maybe I'm in denial when it comes to your cancer," he said, "or maybe I'm so busy being scared about the usual stuff, I haven't even gotten to *that*."

We laughed.

"So what are you saying here?" I asked.

"I'm not sure what I'm saying. I only know that now that it's truly over with Donna, I'm not sure I can handle a man-woman thing."

"How about a boy-girl thing?" I kidded.

"How about a bike ride?"

"Good idea."

We got wine, cheese and bread for a picnic, then rode our bikes to a trail on the mountain that neither of us had ever traveled.

"Look," I said to Michael. "This is uncharted territory."

"I know," he answered. "And it's pretty rocky. Do you think we'll make it?"

"With all we've been through, how bad could it be?"

"Wait a minute," he said. "Are you talking about the trail?"

"*No, stupid*! I'm talking about *us*." Both of us almost fell off our bikes laughing.

"Hey," Michael said, regaining control. "Look over there

at that fire trail; let's go down there and explore."

Down there would mean a big trip *up* later, but I agreed. When we quickly reached a plateau that was both beautiful and totally secluded, with the ocean shimmering in the distance, I said: "I know we've only been riding for two minutes, but is this a perfect place for a picnic, or what?"

"Or what," Michael answered.

"Good. Let's eat."

We emptied our backpacks, cracked open the wine and then, while we sipped, I read to Michael one of my favorite poems, from *archy & mehitabel* by Don Marquis:

the lesson of the moth

i was talking to a moth
the other evening
he was trying to break into
an electric light bulb
and fry himself on the wires

why do you fellows
pull this stunt i asked him
because it is the conventional
thing for moths or why
if that had been an uncovered
candle instead of an electric
light bulb you would
now be a small unsightly cinder
have you no sense
plenty of it he answered
but at times we get tired
of using it

we get bored with the routine
and crave beauty
and excitement
fire is beautiful
and we know that if we get
too close it will kill us
but what does that matter
it is better to be happy
for a moment
and be burned up with beauty
than to live a long time
and be bored all the while
so we wad all our life up
into one little roll
and then we shoot the roll
that is what life is for
it is better to be a part of beauty
for one instant and then cease to
exist than to exist forever
and never be a part of beauty
our attitude toward life
is come easy go easy
we are like human beings
used to be before they became
too civilized to enjoy themselves

and before i could argue him
out of his philosophy
he went and immolated himself
on a patent cigar lighter
i do not agree with him
myself I would rather have

half the happiness and twice
the longevity

but at the same time i wish
there was something i wanted
as badly as he wanted to fry himself

archy

Michael gently tickled my arm. "Kiss me," he said.

"No problem," said I.

Then he began to fumble with my shorts.

"What are you doing?"

"Let's make love."

"Here?"

"Uh-huh."

"Grown-up love? Not high-school love?"

"Yep."

"But isn't this the moment when you're supposed to say, 'Look, I think we should talk about this'?"

"Not anymore."

As we lay on the mountain — the earth our bed, the sky our ceiling, wind our blanket, water our song — I thought: *This* is how my book should end.

Thirteen

❦

But it doesn't. Skip to just a few months later: March 1991, a year and three quarters since my transplant, my forty-fifth birthday on the horizon. I've never been happier. I've never felt healthier. I've never looked livelier. I've never said *die.*

But it's always with me in some small way – like whenever I buy more than one bar of soap, or tickets to a concert three months in advance. In truth, I should have been driven nuts already by my magical thinking – such as, "If I spend like a dying person, I'll live; if I spend like a living person, I'll die." Not to mention the two extremely contrary beliefs that are with me almost every second: that I have somehow, miraculously, marvelously, entirely licked this thing; and that it's only a matter of minutes before I'm totally found out. In other words, at the very same moment I can be absolutely fine and utterly terrified that the cancer is returning to my lungs *right now.* Yet, some-wonderful-

God-knows-how, these contrary thoughts seem to balance each other out – rendering me, at most moments, peaceful, harmonious and as balanced as I've ever known myself to be.

Except when I'm challenged. As on the day in March of '91 when I received, for my approval, an article about my transplant that was to be published in a Nebraska magazine. "She went into the hospital," it said, "and six weeks later, walked out completely cured."

When I read that sentence it was as if someone had put a match to my soul. My whole body began to burn. Sweat poured from my face. I almost threw up; I almost passed out. So superstitious am I, especially with something as mysterious as cancer – MY CANCER – that I was certain the very use of the word *cure* amounted to a death sentence.

I called the writer and ranted at her. "Who ever told you that I've been cured? How dare anyone use that word!" I won't recount the rest of the conversation; suffice it to say that ultimately I summoned my medical records and discovered, much to my surprise, that the doctors with whom she'd spoken had actually declared me in "complete remission." So I allowed her to change the sentence to " . . . six weeks later, she walked out of the hospital, *apparently* in remission."

But believe me, in my double-think way, I was as elated to see the word "remission" in my records as I was nauseated to actually *say* it.

And then . . .

❧

The sun was hopscotching off the Golden Gate Bridge as I drove through the toll gate into the city to interview Dr. Richard Cohen. My hair, finally long enough to flap in the wind, was doing same, thanks to my sunroof. And Van Morrison, singing "So Quiet in Here," was totally wailing on the radio. When I heard the lyric "This must be what paradise is like . . . so quiet in here, so peaceful in here . . ." I burst into if-this-is-as-good-as-it-gets-that's-all-right-with-me tears. So many moments, all so simple. God, do I love it here on earth.

It had been four months since I'd had a routine checkup, and that was on a visit back to Omaha. Now it was time for another checkup, and therefore time to find a local oncologist. Dr. Cohen had been recommended by my acupuncturist/herbalist, so I had a favorable impression already. But I still made it clear, when I scheduled the appointment, that I was new in town and was interviewing doctors.

Cohen's office was messy; I liked that. I also liked his introduction: "Hi. Dr. Dick Jack Cohen here." And I liked it when, referring to my file, at least a foot thick, he asked: "Have you sold the rights to the screenplay yet?"

He took a great history – terrific questions, medical and beyond. He made it clear that he viewed himself and his patients as partners; that if I disagreed with anything he suggested, I should voice it loudly; that he was negotiable. When he prefaced a statement with "If you decide to go with me," I liked that too. In fact, I interrupted him to say, "You just have to pass the physical exam." And I meant it. His hands had to have the professional equivalent of the knowing of a long-time lover. And they did.

In fact – too much. My knowing new doctor found two lumps underneath my right arm.

I told him that one of them had actually been discovered back in 1983 (if, indeed, it *was* the same lump), aspirated with a needle, and found to be benign. After that, it had been followed closely to make sure it didn't get bigger. In 1989, when the cancer recurred, the lump was still there and still the same size. And here it was still.

When I'd seen Dr. Vaughan four months earlier, he too had felt the lump and, at first, had been concerned. When he was reminded that it had been there all along, he was visibly relieved. After all, if it hadn't gotten bigger in all those years, and hadn't gotten smaller either after truckloads of chemo, it seemed highly unlikely to be malignant.

Cohen agreed with this logic. He was concerned, however, by what seemed like a new finding — the *second* lump, a little lower and deeper than the first. Had this second one been missed at my checkup in Omaha? Or had it appeared during the past four months?

"Look," he said. "It's movable; it's on the opposite side from your original cancer; these are good signs, but you never know. My suggestion, and please holler if you disagree, is let's have a surgeon take a look; *I* think it should be biopsied, but let's see what *he* says."

"Take me; I'm yours," I told him. Not only did I love the way he talked, but there was no way I could ignore this finding.

I left the appointment knowing one thing for sure. It was time to spend like a dying person — so I'd live. I went straight to Postrio, one of Wolfgang Puck's finest restaurants, and ate funny food, like sweet and sour quail salad. Then I went to "High Tea" at the Compass Rose in the St. Francis Hotel, where I washed down my quail salad with teacakes and jazz.

Driving back over the Golden Gate Bridge, now socked in by the San Francisco fog, I stroked my hair, wondering how long I'd keep it — yet, strangely, feeling jubilant and free.

First of all, in my deepest gut of guts, I retained a feeling that everything would be O.K. But even when I considered the worst scenario – that this was it; I was dying – I knew I had found the perfect doctor. I knew I was living where I wanted to die.

And I knew that the woman who'd used the word *cure* was responsible for my death.

I am writing this as it is happening – without the benefit of outcome – so that hindsight doesn't blur my truth.

It's the morning before my appointment with the surgeon. I am sitting in my favorite café – inside my body, wrapped in my skin, conscious almost every second of the miracle that I AM HERE. As I watch the people beginning their day, reading their papers, sipping their tea, I wonder who, in this room packed with strangers, will be the next to die. It's always a surprise, never who you expect. Or is it? I wonder, will it be me? My mortality burner is on again. The flame is low; the heat is constant. I am simmering peacefully, bubbling gently, rolling rhythmically, back and forth, dancing between the here and now, the here and then, the here and hereafter . . . the never-again.

Since next week is my birthday, I have made an appointment with a Hindu astrologer to have my "predictive" (how bold of me) chart done. Uncertain as to the exact time of my birth, I spent hours last night in search of my certificate. I never found it; instead I found pictures – scattered photos that, placed in order, formed the history of my hair through ten years of cancer. Fried hair framing yellow skin (1982). Scarved head framing hubcap earrings (1989). Meg Ryan hat framing wigged head (1990). Bald head framing naked soul (also 1990). And finally, a photo taken last week with the Meg Ryan hat over real hair . . . shoulder-length hair, curly, gorgeous, sexy hair, *my* hair (1991). Please, oh, please, I don't want to seem like an absolute pig, but, gosh, I'd *really* like to keep it.

So many feelings. So many thoughts. Part of me up and *living* every day. Part of me on hold – in suspended animation – planning what cigarettes I'll buy if I find out this is it. Then remembering *this was it* two years ago. And I'm still here. How many "this is its" does one person get, anyway? Can I keep on fighting if "this is it" again? My hunch is yes. My hunch is no. One minute I'm thinking *No more treatment, let me finish my book, keep having fun and, as the song says, "live till I die."* The next minute I'm thinking *If only some kind of treatment every few weeks could give me more time – quality time – then I'll live out my months, years, whatever I've got . . . bald head, once again, framing naked soul.*

I can't know what I'll really feel until I learn the truth about the lump. I wish I were sure that if it were malignant I'd refuse further treatment. Because then I wouldn't bother finding out; I'd just live in ignorant bliss. Maybe my answer is hidden in *there*, in the fact that I *can't* say I'd refuse treatment.

I do not feel nervous. Not yet, anyway. Just aware and remembering that limbo time between tests and results . . . between the illusion of forever and the phone call that slams the door. That limbo time where I can still believe I am Ruth Gordon in *Harold and Maude*, living my life to a Cat Stevens soundtrack, making love with a child on my eightieth birthday, dying happy . . . and, most of all, by choice.

I think about the New Age notion that we are responsible for our disease. I waver between embracing it – *oh boy, if we are responsible, I can fix it* – and rejecting it with disgust. When I get real honest, I see that the disgust is directed at myself, or anyway at *part* of me, that all-too-blaming, all-too-addicted-to-perfection part that still believes it *is* my fault. She's littler than she used to be. Which makes, I guess, the rest of me bigger. But she's *still* there. And that's O.K.; I think I can handle her. She just needs love.

So, once again, I'm in that moment of wondering whether to change my name, change my address, pack it up, move to Fiji, fuck my brains out, write my socks off, eat my heart out, smoke my nose off . . . or do my laundry to my favorite soap.

Ah, but these decisions will have to wait. I have an 11:30 appointment for acupuncture with McCulloch. And a 2:00 with Genny, who's warming up those hands as I write.

❧

At McCulloch's – finally, despite my bravado, quiet on the table, with needles in my soul – tears of missing, tears of joy, tears of sadness, tears of life, idle gently down my cheeks.

At Genny's – well, we spend most of the session under my arm.

"It never gets easier, does it?" Dr. Roan, my surgeon, said gently as he met me at the door of the operating room, where my knees were impersonating popcorn popping. We had met the day before and he'd agreed with Dr. Cohen that a biopsy was in order. We would do it under local anesthesia. It would take about an hour. And, thank God, he could fit me in the following day.

Once they got me on the table and covered me with preheated blankets, my knees settled and so did I, which was a relief since I didn't want to take Valium or any other drug that might get in the way of an after-surgery *café au lait* by the Bay.

Everything went smoothly; I hardly felt a thing. And when I did, I would just tell Dr. Roan and he'd give me a little more local anesthesia. As it turned out, the "second" lump might actually have been the "tail" of the first. He said that nothing looked terribly unusual; that nothing was wrapped around anything else; that it looked as good as it could to the naked eye, but we wouldn't know for certain till the pathology report came back the next day.

Minutes after the surgery ended I was hopping into my clothes, alert and eager to do whatever I pleased to pass the torturous twenty-four hours till I'd meet with Roan to discuss the results. The truth, however, was that while a voice in me was saying, "This could be your last day of living in the illusion of 'forever,' better get out there and do something, drink something, smoke something, buy something, fuck something . . ." I really felt like going home, being alone, and just enjoying the view. I didn't even feel like calling Michael.

I didn't feel scared; I didn't feel sad. Tired, yes; but in a state of surrender. If the tumor was malignant, no amount of swimming, visualizing, meditating, praying, bargaining, acupuncturing, swamp-teaing or not eating red meat –

within the next twenty-four hours – could possibly change that fact. So I rested and popped Advil for the pain I was feeling as my arm "thawed out."

Dr. Roan had given me something stronger for the pain, but I didn't want to feel groggy, at least during the day. Before I went to bed, though, I took half of one of the stronger pills. At one point, I awakened to go to the bathroom. The clock said 3:30, so I took the other half, figuring it would help me sleep through the rest of the night. When I returned to the bedroom, however, I discovered I'd misread the clock. The time was actually 6:15. I would've thought that anybody faced with passing the hours till she'd receive a verdict that could change or end her life would welcome a chance to stay unconscious for as much of that time as she could. But *my* reaction went something like: "Shit. I can't believe I *did* that; now I've got to sleep it off and miss the entire morning." There was nothing special I wanted to do; I just wanted to be *awake*.

Watching myself have that reaction was comforting, though. I always look for signs of how I would handle the worst possible news. And this was a clue that I'd want to live fully, no matter how long I had.

I called Michael and told him what was up.

❧

Sitting in the examining room of Dr. Roan's office, in a pale-blue paper gown, I assumed the fetal position and began to shake. Michael was with me. I made him put his ear to the wall and listen to Roan's side of the telephone conversation he was having in the next room.

"Is he talking about me?"

"No, Fanny."

"Are you sure?"

"Yes, Fanny."

"How about now? I think he just hung up and redialed. *Now* he's talking about me, don't you think?"

"No, Fanny." He had tears in his eyes.

Still in the fetal position, I started to rock. Michael put his hand on my back and melted into my rhythm. Then he put his cheek to mine. Under his spell, my thoughts tumbled out.

"I don't know how many more times I can do this – sit here living for that moment when someone opens the door and my eyeballs jump out to meet *his*, to *read his*, to know the answer before he opens his mouth, suffering from the flimsy illusion that if *I* know the answer before he *says* it, *I AM IN CONTROL*.

"I don't know how many more times I can do this – sit here, choreographing my death, planning my funeral, writing my eulogy, missing myself when I'm gone.

"I don't know how many more times I can do this – sit here, almost hoping the tumor's malignant, because as cool as I am most of the time, this is the moment I begin to question whether I can stay this side of sane if I hear the word 'cancer' one more time, and to actually *hear* it and survive *just* the *hearing* would be its own twisted form of relief."

The door opens. The doctor smiles.

"How are your incisions?" he asks.

I have my answer.

Twisted relief.

Fourteen

❦

"I know this sounds crazy," I said to Michael as we left Dr. Roan's office, "but for the strangest reason, this doesn't feel like cooties." We were heading for Dr. Cohen, who had said he'd see us right away.

In 1981, the disease *had* felt like cooties. My first reaction to it was "Get it out of here; take it and take it *now*." And, as with cooties, I couldn't shake the feeling that, even if they removed my entire body, the creepy stuff would *forever* still be there. With the recurrence in 1989, it was even worse, since my cootie theory had been proven valid. So why *now* did I feel strangely calm and optimistic? Was it because when you're living with cancer and always waiting for the other shoe to drop, you feel better once it *has* dropped? Was it because somehow, after all these years, I'd actually, kind of, become "friends" with my cancer? Was it because Genny had said, at our last session, "I think this might be the disease on its way out," and even though

I'd told her no way — that's not how cancer works — on a deeper level, I hoped she was right? Or was it simply a case of complete denial?

Whatever it was, it could quickly be bumped. By the time we sat down with Dr. Cohen, I was hyper, teary, babbling and making extremely bad jokes.

"I'm glad you could see me immediately, Doctor. I'm in a desperate race against time."

"Listen to me, Fanny," Cohen began, trying to reel me back to the planet. "Your last chest X-ray was splendid. Your last bone scan was normal. Your blood work is great. You'll have to have a CAT scan of the chest and another bone scan, just to make sure, but I strongly suspect that the tumor is localized."

"Localized? But isn't my disease considered metastatic? I don't get it."

Cohen went on to explain that, yes, my disease was considered "metastatic," but that if there was no evidence of cancer outside the axillary lymph node area under my right arm, then it wasn't currently "metastatically active." And that — short of having *no* disease at all — was the best circumstance I could hope for. "The biological capabilities of handling it are excellent," he concluded.

"Huh?"

"It's *treatable*, Fanny. Do you understand?"

"What would be the treatment?"

"Assuming there's no evidence of disease anywhere else, surgical removal of the remaining axillary lymph nodes and five weeks of radiation."

"What about chemo?"

"No chemo," he said. "Hormone therapy. Tamoxifen. Just like you've had since after the transplant."

"But doesn't this tumor mean that the Tamoxifen has failed?"

"This tumor has probably been there a long time; the Tamoxifen is most likely what's held it. If there's no evidence of blood-borne, systemic disease, we have to assume the Tamoxifen is still working."

"I'm *so* confused. If the tumor has been malignant all this time, why didn't it respond to high-dose chemotherapy, or conventional chemotherapy, for that matter?"

"Your blood may not have carried the chemo to that area. Or those particular cells might have been resistant to the chemo."

Dr. Cohen could see I was going into overload. He reminded me of what he'd said earlier. I made him repeat it four more times, till finally he wrote it down for me and handed me the paper:

1. Localized.

2. Not metastatically active now.

3. Treatable.

I thanked him, hugged the paper to my heart, and carried it to lunch, where Michael and I celebrated what Cohen had confirmed – it did not feel like cooties. At least, not yet.

❧

My CAT scan and bone scan showed no evidence of disease. My tumor was tested for hormone receptivity and appeared to be even more sensitive than in 1981. This meant that, after surgery and radiation, I'd have a good chance of controlling hormonally any microscopic disease that might have gone undetected.

I was about to call Dr. Vaughan in Omaha to tell him my disease was back, but as it happened he called me first. He wanted to ask if he could give my name to an Associated Press reporter who was doing a series on transplants like mine.

"Sure," I said, "unless he's only looking for people who are in remission."

"What are you telling me?" Vaughan asked.

"Remember that lump under my right arm? The one that was aspirated in 1983 and found to be benign? The one that's probably been there all this time?"

"Oh, no." Vaughan took a deep breath.

"The good news," I told him, "is the tumor appears to be localized."

"That's unusual," he said.

"What do you mean?"

"Well, two things. First, the node was on the opposite side from your original primary; it's not unheard of, but it *is* rare, to have a contralateral recurrence. Second, if this *is* a recurrence of your original tumor, I'd expect it to also have recurred where it did before."

"So what are you saying?" I asked.

"That maybe this is a local metastasis from a *new* primary tumor, in your remaining breast."

"Yikes!" was my sophisticated response. "That would have never *ever* occurred to me."

Vaughan went on, "Without the pathology reports, I'm just guessing, but my hunch is it's from a new primary. When was your last mammogram?"

"Funny you should mention it; Cohen left a message on my machine today telling me to have a mammogram as soon as I can. I figured it was routine, but he must be starting to think along the same lines as you."

"Sounds like it."

"Well, I'm scheduled for a mammogram tomorrow," I told him, "so that'll give us some more information, huh?"

"It should," Vaughan said. "But . . ." He went on to describe further possibilities that left my head whirling. He had seen cases, he said, when a lump had grown from a primary cancer that was literally microscopic in size, or had shrunk away to invisibility. So there might be a new primary even if nothing showed up in the mammogram. Even a comparison of cells from the lump just removed and the one taken out back in 1981 might prove nothing; they might look like cousins and still be from different primary cancers. "In other words," he summed up, "there's no way to ever say definitively that this is *not* from a new primary tumor."

By now I was reeling.

"Actually," Vaughan continued, "it would probably be better if it *is* a new primary."

"Better?" I repeated, puzzled.

"Sure. It would mean your other cancer is still in remission. And a new and different breast cancer *might* have a chance of being cured."

"So what do you suggest I do?" I asked, as I felt myself entering the Twilight Zone.

"I think you should treat this as if it's a new primary tumor."

"You mean even if nothing shows up on the mammogram?"

"Yes."

"And how would that treatment differ from what I'd do for a localized recurrence of the old cancer?"

"Everything would be the same, but you'd also treat the breast."

"What does *that* mean?"

"If nothing shows up on the mammogram, then the best way to get the most information is by having a mastectomy. But you have to ask yourself how you'd feel if even after they've dissected the entire breast, they don't find definitive evidence of cancer." An alternative, he said, would be to include the entire breast, instead of just part of it, in the radiation treatments I would be undergoing in any case. But "the wider the radiation field, the more possible complications, including marrow toxicity, which would *not* be good."

"Well, you've certainly given me a lot to think about," I said, almost out of breath.

"Yeah, I'm sorry."

"Hey, it's your job."

We agreed to talk again, once I got the results of my mammogram as well as my pathology reports. Then I hung up and started praying for the most ridiculous thing I'd ever prayed for: a new primary tumor.

What would be a nightmare to a "normal" person was a ship of hope to me; my mammogram revealed "suspicious microcalcifications." If a biopsy proved they were cancerous, we could assume my original cancer was still in remission and begin to focus on what, to me, by now seemed like a piece of cake – a new and early primary tumor.

But nothing with cancer is ever that easy. The microcalcifications proved to be "normal." Which, as Vaughan had told me, didn't prove there was no microscopic cancer present; it just meant that now I had to decide whether or not to sacrifice my breast in the hope of learning that it was the source of my cancer – and with the awareness that even after the surgery we might *never* know for sure.

The decision came easily. I knew that, no matter how remote the possibility that a new primary tumor was causing my cancer, I would never feel comfortable if we didn't treat my breast. I also knew that I didn't want to, as I called it, "use up my radiation wad" on a field any wider than absolutely necessary. (You can only have a certain amount of radiation to any area of your body.)

So that was *that*. A decade after my first mastectomy, my right breast would join my left, and I would become something I hadn't expected to ever become again – *even*. In a moment when they tell you, "There's something you can do; you can still save your life," it's amazing how easily one can transform a devastating mutilation into a matter of balance.

And a matter of passion. The night before my surgery, Michael and I went to Fleurs de Lys, my favorite French restaurant in probably the world, where we ate everything we could find on the menu that swam. Then, presenting me with a single red rose that he'd plucked from the table, Michael whisked me back to my Bay view haven, where the next ten hours were devoted to tenderly, sweetly, deliciously, gently saying goodbye to my breast.

Whether it was my swamp tea, my acupuncture, my surgeon, or what, my mastectomy and axillary lymph node dissection were way better the second time around. I came back from recovery, at noon, wide awake and stayed that way until midnight. The phone rang soon after I returned to my room. I picked it up to find McCulloch on the other end. Shocked that I was the one who answered, he asked: "Which hand did you use to pick up the phone?"

I looked down, surprised to realize I was already reaching with my operated-on arm.

By the time Michael arrived, I swear, I looked gorgeous. My hair had somehow survived the day and I'd actually had the strength to doll up my face.

The visit was sweet – an endless back rub to a Fred Astaire movie. Then a nice long walk through the hospital halls. Somewhere around midnight, in one of those halls, it occurred to me what had happened that day.

"Oh, my God, Michael. I don't have any breasts."

And bless that boy, without skipping a beat he said, "That's O.K.. I like dark meat."

The facts were in. My breast tissue revealed no evidence of cancer. But my lymph nodes – ten of the thirteen removed – *did*. And the diseased cells looked a lot like the ones preserved from the original mastectomy back in 1981.

So welcome to another episode of "Who Do You Trust?" featuring four fabulous doctors *not* in total agreement.

Behind Doors One and Two – Doctors A and B, who feel it's a contralateral recurrence, meaning the old cancer all over again, although they're not sure if it's actually a recurrence or a "leave behind." Their recommendation: Radiation and continue the Tamoxifen.

Behind Doors Three and Four – Doctors C and D, who feel it's a new primary cancer. Their recommendation: Radiation and switch from Tamoxifan to Megace, the next level of hormonal manipulation.

And who *do* I trust? Whoever it is I spoke with last. Since the truth is – *nobody knows.*

I spent lots of time debating whether to switch to Megace. The details are something of a rat's nest, but I finally decided to stay on Tamoxifen.

Radiation – not to make light of it, but compared to everything I'd already been through – was pretty much a snap.

And since either scenario – a local contralateral recurrence of the old or a local metastasis of a disappearing new – is both quirky and rare, I'd elevated my philosophy about my disease to: "Hey, everybody! It's Mouseketeer Anything-Can-Happen Day!"

❧

Which certainly proved true just a few weeks later, when I was speaking with Michael on the phone one night and, running my hand through my hair, shrieked upon discovering a large lump right on the back of my neck. Fortunately, I was scheduled to see Dr. Roan for a checkup the following day.

"Before you check my mastectomy," I said to Roan, all too many sleepless hours later, "feel this on my neck and tell me it's nothing."

I watched his face as he felt the lump and received my answer in the lines between his brows.

"Shit," I yelled. "Give me a break."

"Look, Fanny. This could be nothing, but with your history, we've got to check it out."

"Surgery?"

"Yes. We can actually do it tomorrow, if you like; I just

had a cancellation."

Why was I never able to get a haircut this quickly? I agreed to the surgery, then pushed Roan to the wall.

"This is bad, isn't it?"

"We won't know till tomorrow."

"O.K., look," I kept going, "if you had to give me a percentage, just a gut-hunch percentage – what are the odds here?"

Reluctantly, this sweet, dear, honest man answered, "My gut hunch? Eighty percent chance it's malignant."

I left, called Michael and said, "Time for the Last Supper."

The question is, how many Last Suppers can you get out of one man? This time, we went to my favorite Italian restaurant, then out to the movies – *Thelma and Louise.* In the end, when Thelma and Louise took their lives by driving heroically into the Grand Canyon, I became hysterical right there in the theatre. Michael held me while I screamed, "Please, I'm not ready; I don't want to die."

And then I said something about my disease I'd never said before. Something that, once I'd said it, I couldn't believe I'd *never said.* Three little words: "It's not fair."

We left the movie and made love in the back seat of Michael's car. What else are you supposed to do before you die? The next day, stretched on the operating table with Roan drilling in the back of my neck, me wondering if I'd have time to finish writing this book, I looked over at the clock, which said 1:29. And just at that moment, sounding as if he'd struck gold, Roan yelled: "This *thing* is a blood clot!"

"I *can* finish my book," I cried.

Everyone applauded. Then they stitched me up and sent

me home, where I checked my machine to discover that at 1:29 *exactly*, my agent, with whom I hadn't spoken in at least six months, had called to ask me, "Where's the book?"

Now if that wasn't "Anything-Can-Happen Day," you tell *me* what is.

PART FOUR

FOR-SAKING THE BEATEN PATH

Fifteen

❦

Time went on. Good things happened, bad things too. The relationship with Michael hit its peak, then declined till finally we parted, still close friends. In my beautiful hillside studio, I wrote and wrote – even though I'd always been afraid, in that magical way I have of thinking, that the minute I finished this book, I'd die.

Twenty minutes after completing what I thought was the final chapter, resting my hand in that space that would be in between my breasts – I found a lump.

Surgery, the next day, revealed a malignancy. A bone scan showed that the tumor had also recurred in my sternum. A CAT scan showed involvement in my mediastinum (the space in the chest between the lungs, breastbone, and spine). And now *all* the doctors agreed that this seemed more like the work of a new cancer than a recurrence of the old – but of course, as always, we would never know for sure.

And, as I looked at the options for treatment, all the "if-then-buts" returned. Plus new ones.

If there was in fact a new primary cancer, perhaps another transplant was in order. I checked it out and the answer was, yes, I *might* be a candidate, but things didn't look good. Although I was probably still in good enough physical shape, my chances of being responsive to chemotherapy were a lot slimmer now, for several reasons. I'd already received several of the "big guns" and had most likely developed resistance to them. Plus, while my cancer was aggressive at the time of my first transplant, it seemed to be slow-growing now. And slow-growing tumors have been shown to be less responsive to chemo than fast ones. Furthermore, this "new" disease had most likely been growing, even if only microscopically, at the time of my first transplant. If it were responsive to high-dose chemotherapy, it probably would have been wiped out then.

All this being true, there was still a small chance I would be sensitive to *some* kind of chemo, but the only way to find out would be to take several courses of a drug I'd never had before, like Cisplatin, and see. Then, if I *did* respond, I'd have to find a transplant program that used higher doses and different drugs than I'd ever had before. No easy task.

Conventional medicine didn't offer me much hope either. There were lots of doctors who would throw me on chemo right away – mainly, I suppose, to be doing *something.* But *my* guys all agreed that, unless I was testing for chemosensitivity with a transplant as my goal, it was time to switch from Tamoxifen to Megace and see if a new hormone might "hold me" for a while. Chemo and radiation, they felt, should be saved for later on, when hormones had failed or when pain management was an issue.

So I switched to Megace and began to wrestle with the weirdness, the guilt, the shakiness, the fear that came with – for the first time in ten years of managing my cancer – *leaving* a stone unturned.

At one point during my deliberations, on the advice of my doctors, I scheduled a pelvic and abdominal CAT scan, plus a bone-marrow biopsy, in order to get more needed information about my transplant eligibility. On the morning of these tests, I found myself thinking about taking Cisplatin. I thought about vomiting. I thought about mouth sores. I thought about fevers. I thought about fatigue. Then I thought about taking the stuff, losing my hair, finding out I wasn't responsive . . . and dying bald.

I called the hospital, cancelled my tests, hung up the phone and said to nobody in particular, "I declare the next twenty-four hours National I-Don't-Have-Cancer Day."

Then, a morning paper and a matinee later, I sat at my favorite outdoor café and tried to figure out what I'd done. I, who was *always* the perfect patient, joking at all the poking and prodding, smiling at all the surgeries and scans, never missing a single appointment, always opting for the biggest gun, forever taking the hugest risk, even when the chances were slim to none – I, who was always the perfect patient, suddenly thought of dying bald and found myself saying, "No!"

Then one day, while at the hospital for a checkup, I noticed a flyer announcing a lecture by Dr. Valentin Ivanovich Govallo, a Russian immunologist whose cancer research I'd actually heard about through some of my more reliable alternative-therapy resources. Govallo would be speaking at the Cancer Support Community, a non-profit center in San Francisco offering tons of wonderful, free cancer help. I had spoken there about my transplant and had become attached, via umbilical phone cord, to the founder, Vicky Wells.

The night of the Govallo lecture, I arrived early so I could get good seats for Vicky and me. Next to me, in the not-Vicky chair, sat a beautiful, reddish-blonde-haired woman with intensely grey/blue/greenish eyes. We each shuffled our papers and got settled. Then she looked at me and zeroed right in on two tiny blue tattooed dots on my neck – a tell-tale sign I'd had radiation (the dots show the technicians where to aim the machine).

"Radiation?" she asked, a swell ice-breaker.

"Yep," I answered.

"Breast cancer?"

"Uh-huh."

"Lumpectomy?"

"Nope."

"Mastectomy?"

"Yep."

"One?"

"No. Two."

"Oh," she lit up. "Washboard!"

I choked. What a gutsy, funny, accurate remark. Though I'd never thought of it, my tight, flat, ribs-on-display chest looked *exactly* like a washboard. And suddenly I knew.

"You must be Nancy Bruning," I said.

"Fanny?" she answered. "Fanny Gaynes?"

Nancy and I had heard of each other through Dr. Cohen

and Vicky Wells. They'd urged us to get in touch – it would be "a match made in heaven." But neither of us had bothered yet. I knew Nancy had written a book, well-known in the cancer world, called *Coping With Chemotherapy*. I'd also heard she was very funny. I hadn't seen how the two went together, until then.

Vicky, Nancy and I struggled through Govallo's lecture, which was, much to our surprise, delivered in Russian, with an interpreter who taught us the true meaning of the phrase "lost something in the translation."

After the lecture, Nancy and I went out for coffee and patched together our meager notes. To sum up: Dr. Govallo's research was based on a similarity between the immune systems of a pregnant woman and someone with cancer. The pregnant woman's immune system doesn't recognize the fetus as a foreign body, and therefore allows it to grow to term. The cancer patient's system doesn't recognize the tumor cells as foreign either, so they too are allowed to grow, with lethal results.

Govallo had developed a treatment designed to prevent the tumor from blocking recognition by the immune system. To the best of our understanding, he used placenta extracts and God-knows-what-else to do this. Once the tumor cells were recognizable, his theory went, the patient's immune system would attack them and kill them. This seemed different to us from most immunological therapies, which attempted to strengthen the immune system but did nothing to change the immunity of the cancer.

Dr. Govallo cited some stunning results from his twenty years of research. True, they weren't controlled studies and the numbers were small, but they included breast cancer and Nancy and I agreed that the theory sounded good. We also agreed that Vicky and Dr. Cohen were right – Nancy and I deserved each other.

No surprise, then, that a month later – when I decided to gamble my life savings on an attempt at saving my life – it was she I chose as the lucky winner of an all-expenses-paid trip to Moscow (since my doctors didn't want me to travel alone).

Sixteen

❦

And now – going totally against everything I'd practiced so far, having no hard data, and more questions than answers – I found myself entering a brand-new era of my cancer management. I like to call it "The Seat of My Pants." My new criteria for what I'd try: (1) No hair loss. (2) Exotic lands.

Nonetheless, putting together the Moscow trip was as Catch-22 as anything else I'd ever done. We couldn't get visas without hotel reservations; we couldn't get hotel reservations without our flights; we couldn't get our non-refundable, non-changeable, difficult to reserve, cheapo flights till we knew we could see Govallo; we couldn't schedule Govallo till we scheduled our flights. And as it turned out, in that special Russian way, the visa office kept us sweating until the last possible hour on the last possible day.

Packing for the trip was yet another story. Dr. Cohen's daughter, Eve, was studying in Moscow, so I asked him to find out what she'd like us to bring in the way of a care package. I expected to hear things like licorice, M&Ms, potato chips, Diet Coke. But after a week of their faxing each other back and forth, Eve finally zeroed in on what she wanted – a few boxes of powdered skim milk and at least a dozen Roach Motels.

For the Russian women who would be handing over their placentas in the name of science, we were to bring lipstick, nail polish, mascara, hosiery and other all-girlie items. We were also advised to bring cigarettes. We hesitated, but, fortunately, sold out in the end; a pack of Marlboros held in a flagging hand could get an otherwise fly-by-you-in-subzero-weather cab to come to a screeching, tail-spinning, ice-slicing halt.

Warned that we might have difficulty finding food, we also packed peanut butter, crackers, trail mix, dried apricots and various other snacks for the swarms of roaches who would be living with us at the Hotel Ukraine – leaving about four inches in each of our suitcases for warm clothing and toiletries.

Ominously, we left San Francisco for the soon-to-not-be Soviet Union on October 20, 1991, the Sunday of the huge Oakland fire. Taking off through dark, threatening clouds of smoke, I couldn't help but wonder: Was this a metaphor for leaving the security of Western medicine? Was I literally burning my bridges behind me?

It took us the entire flight to learn two Russian words, *pahzhahlstah* (please) and *spahsseebah* (thank you), which we promptly forgot the minute we landed in the darkest airport I'd ever *not* seen – a spotlight, every once in a while, hanging from the ceiling – our first Soviet example of *low overhead.*

Driving with our shabby cabbie through the cold, grey, body-gridlocked streets of Moscow, astounded that the Kremlin really looks like the Kremlin, amazed that Red Square really is red, Nancy and I set out on our fairy tale/nightmare in the land of contradictions, where one minute we didn't know where our next meal could be found and the next we were bathing in caviar and cognac.

And then there was Renata – our Russian interpreter/guide/godmother – slightly older than we were, with big, red, bushy hair, eager eyes, extreme intelligence, passion and absolutely no money. Working harder than Nancy and me lumped together, Renata averaged about five American dollars a month. She lived in a very, very dark apartment the size of a hospital room, bursting with papers, books, journals and her bone-thin teenage son, who sat in the dark, strumming his guitar, and refused to let us take him to a restaurant, having never been to one before and worried he wouldn't know how to behave.

Despite it all (or because of it all), Renata always brought us cookies, cakes, teas, flowers (which made us uncomfortable so, of course, we always brought her scarves, gloves, purses, jewelry). And Renata made sure that, amid this potential medical nightmare, we had lots of scattered fun. Thanks to her connections and perseverance, between treatments we made it to the Pushkin Museum; the Hermitage; GUM, the famous department store, where for $1.59 I bought a pair of candelabras that people back home would kill for; and the Army Surplus Store, where I practically got arrested for trying on a uniform. (How was I to know that protocol was to offer a little bribe – pennies, I tell you – to an army official who always just happened to be hovering about, and who had the authority to purchase a treasure or two?) I came away with a perfectly fabulous Soviet belt buckle, complete with a "that'll-never-do" belt, for under two bucks (plus air fare, hotel, food, expenses, gifts, emergencies, but hey . . .).

(Renata also got us to the circus, but there are no words, English or Russian, to describe that smelly, unprofessional, depressing, truly-from-another-time-and-place event. At the other end of the scale, she got us into the Bolshoi. But, alas and alack, it wasn't exactly "ballet" night, per se; more like pilot night at NBC – with a pilot that never made it to prime time. The sets and costumes were magnificent, though.)

On my first day of treatment, Renata and a "driver" friend picked up Nancy and me in plenty of time, but an unexpected taxi strike kept us nervously gridlocked for most of the trip, leaving no time to stop at the American Medical Service to buy disposable needles as we had planned. Many had warned us of the unsanitary, often archaic medical methods in Russia. I wasn't about to turn around at this point, however, so I gave my shoulders a Russian Roulette shrug and planned my memorial service once again. ("The beauty of it was she didn't die of cancer; it was needles that got her in the end . . ..")

Visiting Dr. Govallo's clinic was like dropping into the set of a World War II movie. Sitting in the dark, barren waiting area, I was unnerved by watching a young, babushka'd mother hugging her daughter the way one might hug a child-sized cactus, trying to avoid a weird, invisible, brace-like device that was causing the little girl's pleated skirt to hang like an umbrella destroyed by the wind.

To my relief, no under-the-skirt contraptions were awaiting me in Govallo's clinic. Just a sweet, impassioned doctor, a devoted, gold-toothed "medical sister," and a serum-filled comedy-show prop of a syringe that was so big it made me look thin.

Dr. Govallo tested my blood in a sectioned plate. My memory of this is vague, but each section held a glob of a different color (one, in particular, looked like Gerber's strained peas) and my blood got mixed with each glob to give him the information he needed. Next I got my big, big, huge, huge placenta-and-whatever shot, which burned like honeymoon cystitis of the leg, but was over more quickly, thank God.

After treatment number one, we were free for three whole days, so Nancy and I zipped off to our local travel agency to see about a jaunt to St. Petersburg. As I relate what unfolded, I beg you to remember the life-and-death context in which it occurred.

Mutnick Travel Agency was an eight-by-eight-foot room in the Hotel Belgrade, where we stayed when a convention got us booted out of the Ukraine. (The Belgrade had great all-you-could-eat breakfasts for about four cents – if you didn't mind cockroaches dancing on your grits.)

Mutnick's was decorated mainly in ashtrays. In Russia, no one *doesn't* smoke at any given time. Yet, as if in a movie, when we opened the door the haze somehow, miraculously, lifted, revealing Uri Zvi Levi Chaim Mutnick – Owner, Entrepreneur and Stud Extraordinaire. I mean Uri had teeth. Uri didn't smell. Uri didn't have stains on his pants. Uri was Jewish. Born in Kiev. My mother would be thrilled. It must be love.

And all the stars were in alignment. That evening – the

very same evening when Nancy and I wanted to take the night train to St. Pete's – Uri also needed to go there, for a meeting to be held the next morning. The three of us arranged to have dinner together, after which Nancy and I would be personally escorted by Mr. Hunkeroo to our exciting destination. And not to worry about a thing; Uri would make all the plans.

The dinner/nightclub he took us to was straight out of a really bad movie. Huge was the operative word. Everyone except the three of us was dressed in sequins, with lots of powder-blue and plenty of what appeared to be actual wedding clothes.

We started with cognac. And never stopped. The red caviar, for some reason, tasted better than their black and way better than the red as we knew it back in the States. So we oinked it up on that for quite a while. Then Uri offered to order us a salad, which made me moan in delight, having missed lettuce desperately since we'd arrived in Russia. Their version of salad, however, is a "Conehead"-shaped, mayonnaise-infested mountain of potato salad. It comes with even more mayo drizzled all over it in rivulets, like hot fudge on an ice cream sundae. I looked at this potato pile and thought "Never!" By the end of the trip, though, it was all that I craved. When in Rome. When in Moscow. When insane.

In between live acts that Ed Sullivan would have adored, Uri and I danced and I whispered in his ear, trying to explain to him, to no avail, why it was funny that they were playing "Feelings," not to mention a disco version of "Itsy Bitsy Teenie Weenie Yellow Polka Dot Bikini."

❧

The train ride was quite romantic. The three of us

shared an ancient, forest-green compartment, where we were served scrumptious Russian tea in glass cups with silver holders that had Russian historical scenes on them.

We sipped and talked till we couldn't anymore. Then we closed the blinds and hunkered down for the night, Nancy on one side of the compartment and Uri and me on the other. All our possessions were piled on a table in the middle of the floor. There were no beds and the seats were so skimpy that all of us scrambled and fidgeted for the longest time, till we finally found comfortable positions. Mine was on top of Uri, supported by a most surprising hint of a bulge.

Now that we were all settled, it was pitch-black and so quiet that I actually forgot Uri and I weren't alone. His air mattress grew, along with my desire. Before I knew it, our hands were defining our faces in the dark. Blind love. My little Chicken Kiev. Dream-like and drunken, we squirmed and hugged and kissed and rubbed. When he began to unpeel me, my mind tuned in to Radio Slut.

What are you doing? Are you nuts or what? You don't even have condoms. And you know how empty you've always felt after an evening of too-soon sex.

But this might be different. He comes from the homeland of your people's people. His hair is so soft. His lips are so gentle. Maybe you're soulmates. Part of the same star . . . split at birth.

I refused to let Uri Mutnick unpeel me. But that didn't stop me from unpeeling *him.* My ripe banana in the middle of the night. Monkey business. Primitive abandon. Forget about AIDS. What was I thinking? Oh, well . . . When in Rome. When in Moscow. When insane.

And then – like the brightest bolt of lightning I'd ever

seen, the doors of the compartment flew open, revealing me and – oh, my God, who *is* this man from Kiev upon whom I'm writhing anyway?

I was certain I was being arrested for sex – until I heard Nancy guffawing. It was she who had opened the door, to go find the bathroom. It was she who, thanks to her impeckerable timing, saved me from a disastrous life as Mrs. Fanny Mutnick.

My second and third treatments with Dr. Govallo went smoothly. The only side effects were a little fatigue, a lot of soreness at the site of the injection, a slight fever, and that was that.

To celebrate my third and final treatment, we had Renata pick us up some globby meat, potato-salad mountains, cakes, cookies and wine. And there in the office, amid its barren, impoverished, antiseptic atmosphere, the medical sisters whipped out a gorgeous lace tablecloth, lace napkins, exquisite teacups, plates and wineglasses, all of which felt like treasures that had been hidden for hundreds of years. About ten of us, including Dr. Govallo, sat around the beautiful, warm table, chatting in no known broken language, yet somehow communicating, through spirit, our love and hopes for one another. It is truly my sweetest memory of Russia.

So . . . after three excruciating syringes full of voodoo, plus ten adventure- and cockroach-filled days, I mailed a postcard to the folks back home: "Oh my Godskee, what am I doing *here?* Food fabulous. Shopping divine. Treatment successful; my breasts grew back. XXOO." Then we returned to the U.S. to wait for the magic to kick in.

Seventeen

❦

The good news was . . . three months later, a bone scan of my body and a CAT scan of my chest revealed stable and in some spots regressed (perhaps Govallo really worked?) disease. The *bad* news, however, was . . . while they were looking, they just happened to notice that my right kidney was completely "shut down" and my left one was on its way.

It was time for a pelvic and abdominal CAT scan – the very test I'd so frivolously cancelled when I declared "National I-Don't-Have-Cancer Day." The test for which I now had no baseline, in case there *was* disease.

Which, of course, there was. In my abdomen. *And* my pelvis – twisted around, and squeezing off, my right ureter, the little pipeline between the kidney and the bladder. And with no symptoms and no baseline, I had no idea whether this was brand-new and growing or whether it had been there a long time and was stable or regressing, like my other "stuff." I did know that, old or new, it was *now* threatening major organs.

So the quest continued, the battle raged on, I journeyed farther into Cancerland. And that process continues as I write.

On the advice of Dr. Cohen, I went to a urologist who protected my kidneys by surgically (through my urethra ... ouch) inserting "J stents," teeny plastic tubes that re-opened the ureters. Then, lo and behold, my new and bullish criteria for treatment – no hair loss and exotic travel – went right down the toilet as I traipsed off to Denver to interview for probably the only program in the world that would even consider someone in my condition a candidate for a *second* transplant.

As it turned out, Denver was willing to accept me as a candidate, but without any predictions at all concerning toxicity levels, my chances of responding and the durability of the response, if any. I would be one of the first to go through the program. They were using higher doses than they'd ever used before, and the nickname for one of the drugs they were using, BCNU, was "Be see'n you."

Needless to say, I had a lot of trouble getting excited about the program. But I allowed it to haunt me as a possibility while I reverted to leave-no-stone-unturned mode and proceeded to spend the next two months – non-stop, beyond full-time – calling across the country, calling across the *world*, investigating every clinical breast-cancer trial I could get my telephone mitts on, from Japanese vaccines (made from your own urine) to extracts of shark cartilage. (Did you know sharks are the only animals that never get cancer?)

The problem (to put it lightly) was that at this point, according to statistics, if I didn't have conventional chemo I'd live less than a year; one doctor even said less than six months. Yet, in order to leave no stone unturned, I needed to investigate the clinical trials *before* resorting to conventional chemo, since chemotherapy might preclude me from the trials.

To confuse things more, I knew just how much enthusiasm I would have to muster in order to offer myself up for treatment – *any* treatment, even conventional chemo.

For the first seven weeks, as I called and researched and discussed and brooded over plan after plan and nothing got me even close to a buzz, the one thing that kept me sane was knowing I retained the option to say "no" . . . to it all.

The flip-side of this was that, knowing I might ultimately refuse to choose *any* treatment, I resented the possibility that my research was eating up two precious months of the few I might have left.

By the eighth week, thank God, somewhere between urine and sharks, I learned of two programs that sounded thrilling to me. Both would take me in a new direction. I'd had extensive experience of the three main modalities of conventional cancer treatment, surgery, radiation and chemotherapy; now I could investigate a fourth – biological therapy.

Both programs would make use of my own tumor tissue. In one of them, at an institution in Tennessee, the tissue would be incubated in a laboratory with Interleukin-2, a recently discovered compound that can stimulate certain blood cells into increased anti-cancer activity. If these "killer cells" could then be successfully cultured, they would be reinfused into my body in hopes of shrinking the cancer. The second program, in Newport Beach, Calif., worked along somewhat similar lines; there, technicians would cultivate the tissue in hopes of growing a vaccine specific to my tumor.

While both programs had had promising results with some cancers, such as melanoma and kidney, it was still too early to make breast-cancer predictions. Until recently, the Tennessee program had had a difficult time growing the Killer Cells from breast-cancer tissue. New technology seemed to have improved the chances; still, there were no guarantees. And the folks in charge of the Newport Beach program warned me that they too had had trouble with breast-cancer tissue. But they were willing to do a study of mine, just in case.

Well, all of this was right up my alley. Treatment that theoretically made sense to me . . . with less available data than even my recent rendezvous in Russia. Exciting, adventurous, cutting-edge, with enough unknowns to provide for me my favorite elixir . . . mystery/hope.

It was the Tennessee program that I found most inviting, and two friends I had made along the Cancer Road helped open the door to it. One was Michael Broffman, the master of the Pine Street Clinic in San Anselmo, that wonderful place for acupuncture and herbs and endless support that had helped draw me to Marin County. The other was Vicky Wells, head of the Cancer Support Community in San Francisco. It was they who turned me on to Dr. Robert K. Oldham, founder and director of the Biological

Therapy Institute in Franklin, Tenn.

Dr. Oldham had worked with the National Cancer Institute in researching how the body's own disease-fighting systems might be turned against cancer. Later, back in private practice, he'd created an organization called the National Biotherapy Study Group, whose members work cooperatively on clinical trials of biotherapy methods. I was impressed with his credentials, and even more when I discovered that he also registers an eleven on the humanity Richter.

Dr. Oldham, contacted by Vicky, said he indeed had a program that might be of value to me, but suggested I first call the National Cancer Institute; they had a similar program, he said, and theirs would be entirely free, even to the inclusion of airfare, meals and hotel. So Vicky and I, using conference dialing, spent a long, frustrating session listening to recordings and being referred around the institute's bureaucracy, only to finally reach an administrator who devoted at most forty-five seconds of his valuable time to assessing my case and ruling me out. The NCI didn't want to deal with kidney complications.

To tell you the truth, I was relieved to be rejected. Free treatment would have been impossible to turn down, but my gut was already convinced that Oldham was my guy.

❧

On the plane to Nashville, I mentioned to the flight attendant that my stomach was a bit upset.

"Then you shudenoughta have the leesagna fer lunch."

I said I had some bouillon cubes and asked for a cup of hot water.

"Well, right now I'm beezy as a bumblebee in a bucket of tar, but I might could hep ya in a spell or two."

I began to wonder if I was going to need a translator in Tennessee as well.

The Biological Therapy Institute turned out to be a comfortable, modern, two-story building, housing not only Dr. Oldham's offices but a company that published magazines for cancer patients and professionals. It was just a few minutes' walk from the Williamson Medical Center, where I would go for any parts of my treatment requiring hospitalization.

In fact, if it turned out I was indeed a candidate for the institute's program, the Williamson people and I would be getting to know each other right away. This was because both Oldham's program and the California one required that the tumor tissue I supplied be good and fresh. So I was facing what would essentially be major *elective* stomach surgery.

During the weeks before my arrival, I had tried to come up with as many reasons as I could to justify such extensive voluntary torture. I'd settled on five of them, in this order of importance:

1. To verify that the tumor had actually spread from my breast cancer – that it wasn't from an entirely new primary cancer.
2. To get enough tissue for Dr. Oldham's program.
3. To send the remainder to the vaccine program in Newport Beach.
4. To send anything left after that to Oncotech, a lab in Irvine, Calif., for a chemosensitivity assay. This was a relatively new kind of study that could help determine a person's probability of responding to chemo therapy.
5. Simply to get as much cancer out of me as possible.

Well, indeed I was a candidate, and indeed I went through torture. But I had no idea it was torture until two weeks later, when the Demerol wore off and I flew back to San Francisco with wire loops holding my stomach together and making me look like a shar-pei dog.

Now began a period of waiting to see if my cells would kindly cooperate with the Tennessee lab technicians and multiply into the billions.

Under the program – known as TDAC, for Tumor-Derived Activated Killer Cells – my tissue was being cultivated along with Interleukin-2 in hopes of stimulating the growth of T-lymphocytes, white blood cells that have natural anti-tumor reactivity. Presumably, the T-lymphocytes found in my tumor had already developed a mechanism to combat the cancer, but on their own they could not succeed because the cancer cells outgrew and overwhelmed them. But if a great quantity of Killer Cells could be grown in the laboratory, then reinfused in my body, the theory went, then perhaps they'd have better odds against the disease. To help them in this mission, the Killer Cells would be accompanied on re-entry by interferon and more Interleukin-2.

Growing the Killer Cells was expected to take about six weeks. During that time, Dr. Oldham wanted me to have as much chemotherapy as I possibly could, in hopes of shrinking the cancer or, at least, preventing any new growth. Results of the chemosensitivity assay had come in and indicated that I still had a "relatively good chance" of responding to chemotherapy. Excellent news since, with all the prior treatment I'd had, my chances were getting slimmer.

So, once again, I gathered together a zillion scarves, hats and a wig in preparation for "fallout" and began treatment with Dr. Cohen.

Chemo wasn't too bad this time. There's a new drug called Zofran that, administered with chemo, can prevent nausea *and* keep you lucid. I actually went out for dinner after some of my treatments, a heretofore unheard-of possibility. And my hair thinned a little, but never vanished altogether. Plus, I had the company of another of my wonderful friends for life, Diana Grand – childhood playmate, college roommate, traveling companion and longtime personal crisis counselor – who lived in Berkeley and came to be with me during the treatment.

Several weeks into chemo, I got the great news that my cells had "taken off" – started to grow like gangbusters – and would soon be waiting for me in cryopreservation. I also got word that the tissue sent to Newport Beach had indeed produced a vaccine. I was so excited. It made turning myself into a shar-pei dog worth every wrinkle and every growl.

The question now was timing. We evaluated the benefit of my chemo after six rounds and found the results were pretty good: The tumor hadn't shrunk, but it hadn't grown any either. Dr. Oldham felt that now was the optimum time to try the TDAC program.

In my usual cool-exterior-but-what-a-mess-underneath way, I was excited, scared and desperately in need of immediate consumer therapy. I went to a second-hand store and found the perfect items: Two pair of men's rayon drawstring pajama bottoms from the forties. One was a fabulous paisley in just my colors – rust, green, maize, etc. The other was green with scads of white birds on the diagonal, kind of like an M.C. Escher painting. Anyway, they could be worn as totally hip slacks or as hospital PJs – which reminded me of those "Day to Night" Barbie dolls where her lovely professional working-girl ensemble just needed a boa-like pink thing snapped to the hem and she'd be ready for a va-va-va-voom night with Ken. Mine would just be the reverse: Check in wearing hip contempo pants, dyno blouse, killer jacket, earrings to my knees (Rule 1: The shorter the hair, the longer the earrings), and in seconds be sporting plain old men's drawstring pajamas and a chestful of catheters with tubes twisted around a heavy, double-decker, impossible-to-walk-with pole.

My friend Diane Levine, the producer who had scraped me off the floor when I had my first recurrence four years back, accompanied me to Tennessee. We'd allowed a little extra time for relaxing and sightseeing before my hospital check in, but it turned out we had three full weeks for recreation because there had been an unanticipated delay in producing my Killer Cells.

At first we thought we'd just relax, check out Franklin (after all, it's a Civil War town – it ought to have some interesting Civil War jewelry), then travel, perhaps to the Smokies, maybe even fly to New Orleans. The travel plans moved into first place after we found that the cottage I'd rented sight-unseen was flooded, owing to a broken water heater, and the company that came to clean up the mess decided to forestall mildew by spraying the place with Tutti Frutti – that special smell that gets your patrons in and out of restrooms in a flash.

Diane and I packed as quickly as we could and left town. But we were back in almost no time, because shortly after enduring a ghastly smorgasbord in Gatlinburg, Tenn., I got sicker than I'd ever been to that point in my entire charmed life.

Getting so sick, at a time when I wanted to be as strong as possible for treatments, scared the rest of our travel plans out of me. Instead, Diane and I hung around Franklin, bought a lot of incense and potpourri to overcome the Tutti Frutti, and made little day excursions to Nashville (half an hour away) or local movie theaters. The one in downtown Franklin actually served hot dogs, chili, wine and chips. Life was good again. No complaints.

By the time my cells were ready, Diane had gone back to Los Angeles and my old friend Steffie had arrived. So she and I had the honor of being with each other during my first biological therapy treatment. Owing to the pre-medication, I don't remember much. I *do* remember a plastic bag filled with what looked like a huge batch of sperm, all creamy, sticky and winter white. Those were my Killer Cells? Go, cells!

I also remember thinking I should be doing something highly spiritual while they flowed through my body. After all, as it turned out, I was the first person *ever* to have exactly this treatment for breast cancer. Whether you went in through the "high-tech" door or the "first-ever" door, this was no small moment. I tried to listen to some New Age music, but it didn't do the trick. What did was Van Morrison, Joe Cocker and Eric Clapton.

The treatment lasted five days, pumping me full of Killer Cells, Interleukin-2 and interferon. At first I felt rough and tough and not very sick at all. As the days went on, however, it turned as difficult as, if not worse than, any treatment I'd ever had. The most devastating effect was an indescribable fatigue that left me rolled up in a noodle-ball at the bottom of my bed. Couldn't move. Couldn't mo . . . Cou . . .

❧

After four of these treatments, we paused to evaluate their effect on me. We were hoping the tumor would be smaller now; if so, we would do four more "maintenance" treatments using Interleukin-2 and interferon, but no cells.

Unfortunately, the tumor had not diminished. On the other hand, it hadn't grown, and that meant I could now be considered "stable."

When you're dealing with cancer, "stable" is nothing to sneeze at. And that gave me an excuse, finally, to employ an expression I'd learned from someone at the institute the very day I was admitted for treatment. When Dr. Oldham asked me how I felt about being stable, opportunity hurled it from my otherwise dainty mouth.

"How do you 'spect I feel, Doc? I'm as happy as a two-dick dog!"

Oldham, a true Southern gentleman, acquired an immediate sunburn that lasted two weeks.

❧

If you've ever spent a year more *in* the hospital than *out*, you'll understand the difference an incredible nursing staff can make in the quality of each day and each long night. The extraordinary nursing staff on the oncology floor of Williamson Medical Center is a tribute to the nursing profession. As much as any medication they ever gave me, it was their professionalism and kindness that kept me going.

One night, one of my nurses caught wind of the fact that the following day I was expecting a visitor. She knew my company was six-foot-three. She knew my company had a moustache.

Sometime in the middle of the night I felt a delicious breeze flutter across my toes. I was sure I was dreaming till I opened my eyes and was blinded by a flashlight. It was my nutso night nurse spiffing me up with the pedicure of my dreams.

After the fourth-treatment evaluation, Dr. Oldham thought I should continue the Interleukin-2 on the possibility that it had contributed to my stable status. He also suggested that I add an experimental chemo to the mix – Taxol, the new drug derived from the yew tree about which there had been so much recent hoopla.

Since I dreaded going through the first couple of treatments alone, it was time to call in the troops. But their ranks were thin. My mother couldn't come, because my father was extremely ill and could not be left alone. My sister Carol also was involved in his care. And my sister Mindy had recently added an infant to her family, making it impossible to get away for longer than two days.

Enter Aunt Flo.

This aunt of mine is seventy-five, looks fifty, is gorgeous, and I mean gorgeous – stunning face, beautiful curly white hair, great body, with more energy than I ever had, bright, funny, hip, cultured. The only problem – she saves string.

Nonetheless, it was decided that Aunt Flo would come stay with me for a few weeks. The place was big. There was room for string.

For me, memories came rushing back: When I was six my parents were out of town and I came down with the flu.

Aunt Flo visited every day, soothing me with that sweet, gentle, easy voice that was as beautiful singing as it was speaking, crooning forties songs that are still a part of my soul. And every day she brought me a perfect gift. (My favorites were those sewing cards that you laced yarn through. Aunt Flo tried to persuade me to save excess yarn, but you could already see a rebel in the making.)

Aunt Flo insisted on staying overnight at the hospital and, I'll tell you, somebody forgot to unwire her from motherhood; she was great to have around. I could be in a preconscious state of considering a cough and she would fly up from her bed asking, "What do you need?"

I made it though the first Interleukin-2 and Taxol treatment without much incident, and after a few days we were free to go back to the cottage, thank God no longer smelling of Tutti Frutti. The weather was getting warmer and my landlords had a pool, plus a lovely, gardened backyard. Aunt Flo and I spent some gorgeous days outside, reading, talking, listening to music and eating tuna melt (with soy cheese, of course) al fresco.

One day, " 'laxin' " in the sun, I was reading some of the literature on side effects from the Taxol box (do I know how to have fun?) when suddenly three words screamed off the page: "COMPLETE HAIR LOSS."

Now, I hadn't expected to get away with murder here. Doctors, nurses and consent forms had warned me, and I knew I would be losing some hair. But this was the first time I'd seen "COMPLETE" attached to the concept of hair loss. I was horrified. Then thoughtful.

I recalled the only other time I'd lost all my hair – back in 1990, when *exactly* two weeks after chemo began my hair fell out in eight huge clumps. And a Great Idea came to me.

"Aunt Flo," I hollered. "How are you at giving haircuts?"

"Slightly better than I am at pulling teeth."

Comforted, for some unknown reason, I started to tell her my plan. "Listen, Aunt Flo, remember how cute my hair looked that time it all fell out – when I still had curls and tendrils to pull down from under my hats?" She did. "Well, here's the idea. Before any *more* hair falls out – while I've still got some *control* here – I want a special haircut. Kind of a reverse job."

"I want to leave my real bangs and tendrils and cut off everything else."

"Everything *else?!*"

"So we can use my *own* hair from on top to make as many tendrils as we can. We'll use tape to tie up each one at the top . . . like a bunch of little pony tails."

"Pretty clever," Aunt Flo said. And now she was getting excited. Before I knew it, I was alone by the pool and Aunt Flo was puttering in this little greenhouse area to the side of our cottage. Minutes later she returned with, I swear, a huge pair of garden shears and some big black electrical tape.

Aunt Flo took a swipe. Then six more mighty chops – this time much nearer to the skull. Then she took a hank of hair she had snared and wrapped it lovingly with electrical tape. When she held it up, you could just tell that it would look great taped to the inside rim of my favorite hat, hanging sexily down the nape of my neck.

We had run out of available hair, but now we had a lovely box of electrically taped tendrils. Tendrils-in-waiting – just waiting for the moment when my hair would fall out in huge clumps.

But wait a minute! As I stared into the mirror at my oddly tonsured head – bearing a fringe of wavy locks around a short, rough shag – a ghastly realization came. I looked like I was playing the lead role in the commercial for the Hair Club. It was hat-and-scarf time – *I needed those tendrils now!* And then something else dawned on me – what if I wasn't going to lose any more hair *at all?*

When I got around to asking the nurses, all said they'd never known a patient to suffer complete hair loss from Taxol – and I never did lose all my hair!

Eighteen

❦

Every time I shut my eyes and try to visualize heaven, all I come up with is a bunch of clouds surrounding a fifties Airstream diner. My dad's at the counter eating all the fried food he couldn't eat on earth. His brother Ernie is next to him eating all the fried food *he* couldn't eat on earth. And my grandma's behind the counter frying all the same foods she used to fry on earth anyway.

I'm off at a jukeboxed table listening to Buddy Holly, nursing a double-chocolate milkshake, chain-smoking a pack of filterless Camels, and writing my latest book, *Why Would I Wanna Find a Man if I'm Alive?*

Around 10 every morning Joni's dad comes in to eat a huge piece of apple pie and give his daily report on Joni. Although George has been here several months now, he's still totally aware of every move Joni makes. The good news today is that she and her husband, Charlie, have purchased another dog; they're thinking of naming him Fanny. The bad news is: The silver leafing in the condo is peeling like foil off a Juicy Fruit wrapper, her car phone is broken, they're out of soy cheese at the grocery and her shirts have come back from the dry cleaner's without enough starch in the Victorian collars.

I can't imagine anything worse than dealing with the death of one of your children. On April 21, 1993, after more than a decade of horrible health, my father, Boris Francis Gaynes, died. My first, overriding response was: "Thank God he didn't live to see *me* die." Never was I more certain of the proper order of things.

But why haven't I cried yet? *Not one tear.* Is it simply the comfort of knowing that when he finally went, he went in peace? Is it my own need to see death as an O.K. process? Is it that I'm afraid if I start, I'll never stop? All of the above? Some of the above? I'll cry when I'm ready? Probably a bit of everything.

Three weeks before my father died, I celebrated my forty-seventh birthday. At the party I was surrounded by girlfriends who go back as far as third grade. As we stuffed our faces with designer cuisine, sang oldies to a crackling karaoke machine, and called ex-boyfriends across the nation, I remembered back to my forty-third birthday, when Joni, Marilyn and I named ourselves "The Pointless Sisters." I couldn't help but ask myself how I'd been so lucky as to make it to this day. Physically, of course, I know that lots and lots of medical treatment has helped keep me here on the planet. But what about the emotional side? People are always asking.

There are two gifts I got from working with Brugh Joy that altered my perception of emotional wellness. For years I'd believed that mental health could be attained by finding out what aspects of yourself didn't make you happy and getting rid of them. To Brugh, this notion was self-defeating: He said it was like the way a child "fixes" the pegs in his workbench by hammering them until they're even with the surface of the bench. They're all still there, though, on the other side. From him I began to learn a new way of looking at those parts of me I'd been wanting to pound out of view.

The second lesson was even more important. Before Chicago, my big concern with my disease was what if I die, what if I die, what if I die. As my work with Brugh helped me let go of that fear, a larger question became clear: What if I live?

One night in a dream I wrote:

What if I live and have to awaken every day to sunrise skies?

What if I live and have to awaken every day to hug the trees that hug me back and climb the mountains to take a nap wrapped inside the dogs?

What if I AWAKEN and have to live every day to bathe with the insects and make love with life?

No, I don't know what the dogs and insect baths are about, but the dream did tell me I didn't simply want to "not die" – I wanted to *live.*

That's the real reason I've fought so hard. That's what supplied me with the energy, the spirit, to keep on going.

It was after the transplant, Brugh Joy, and the dream that I started to write this book. Somehow they gave me the confidence to believe that the lessons I've learned are valuable ones to impart.

So if ever any of you are in my situation:

1. Develop a style that is true to yourself, or as Quentin Crisp said: If you discover that you are a bore, don't be *just* a bore – be a *crashing* bore.
2. Don't be nervous thinking you're supposed to live every day *really* trying to smell every flower. Because it's a full-time job with a lot of pressure, and who are we kidding – not all of them smell great.
3. If you're concerned about dying young, try something normally reserved for older folks. My favorite: Putting on lipstick – crooked – while looking into a cracked mirror in a tearoom around 3:00 in the afternoon.
4. If everyone who had stress in their life got cancer, everyone would have cancer. You are not guilty. You are not to blame. These things happen.
5. You don't have to have all your parts fixed to be whole.
6. Become as portable as you can. The resources you need to enrich your life are available no matter where you land.
7. Be wise enough to realize that some people vanish because they just can't handle it, not because they necessarily love you less.
8. If your life should feel smaller, be aware of how delicious even the teeniest things can be.
9. Dump the need to stay perky and entertaining – or stoic and uncomplaining, if that's your model in-

stead. Letting others give to you can be your way of giving to them.

10. Forgive people for being who they are and not who you need them to be. Call ex-spouses, scared friends and those who ran away and let them know it's O.K.. Remember, though, this is for *you*, not for them, so if it doesn't feel right, don't do it.

❧

Just last week I made a call to Alex, the one who said, "I'm sorry *I'm* not dying of cancer, but I have problems too." It was Yom Kippur, the holiday of repentance and forgiveness. The conversation went like this:

Alex: "Hello?"

Fanny: "Alex! Fanny Gaynes."

Alex: "Well, Fanny Gaynes."

Fanny: "So how are you doing?"

(Fifteen unbearable seconds of silence.)

Fanny: "So that's it?"

Alex: "Yup." CLICK. DIAL TONE.

"How am I gonna to find a man if I'm dead?"

I think it'll be a lot easier.

On Oct. 31, 1993, Fanny Gaynes joined her father at the Airstream Diner. If Fanny were writing this epilogue, she would not want that date to be remembered, but rather each day that went before, which she lived to the fullest and shared to the fullest with those she loved.